HEALTH POLICY AND POLITICS

For Peter, Jessica, Amy and Ben
(and Fin and Flora)

Health Policy and Politics

Edited by

ALISON HANN
University of Wales, Swansea, UK

ASHGATE

Published by
Ashgate Publishing Limited
Gower House
Croft Road
Aldershot
Hampshire GU11 3HR
England

Ashgate Publishing Company
Suite 420
101 Cherry Street
Burlington, VT 05401-4405
USA

Ashgate website: http://www.ashgate.com

British Library Cataloguing in Publication Data
Health policy and politics
1. Great Britain. National Health Service 2. Medical policy - European Union countries 3. Medical policy - Great Britain
I. Hann, Alison
362.1'0941

Library of Congress Cataloging-in-Publication Data
Health policy and politics / edited by Alison Hann.
p. ; cm.
Includes bibliographical references and index.
ISBN 978-0-7546-7064-3 (hardback : alk. paper)
1. Medical policy--Great Britain. 2. Medical care--Political aspects--Great Britain. I. Hann, Alison.
[DNLM: 1. Great Britain. National Health Service. 2. National Health Programs--organization & administration--Great Britain. 3. Delivery of Health Care--organization & administration--Great Britain. 4. Health Policy--Great Britain. 5. Politics--Great Britain. WA 540 FA1 H396 2007]

RA395.G6H4235 2007
362.10941--dc22

2007020563

ISBN: 978 0 7546 7064 3

Printed and bound in Great Britain by MPG Books Ltd, Bodmin, Cornwall.

Contents

List of Figures and Tables

Figures

Tables

Notes on Contributors

Arturo Alvarez-Rosete is Health Policy Researcher at the London-based foundation the King's Fund. Arturo holds a PhD in Politics from the University of Nottingham (UK) and has been a visiting lecturer at several universities in Europe and Latin America. Arturo specialises in public policy and public administration, with particular interest in the structures of government and governance and the policy process in health. He is currently working on developing best practice models for health policy making and on international comparisons of health regulatory systems.

Nick Boyd Joined the Department of Health (DH) in the UK in 1977 after studying History and German at Oxford University, and teaching in Germany. He has held a number of policy jobs in DH in public health, health and social care. He went on secondment to the German Ministry of Health in 1981 and again in 1991, working on EU policy there. From 1993–6 he was secretary to the top management board of DH, and from 1999–2006 he was Director of International Affairs. During this time he oversaw the health component of the UK's Presidency of the EU. He was a member of the EU High Level Committee on Health and the High Level Group on Health Services and Medical Care, and part of the UK delegation to the World Health Assembly. Nick is currently on a year's sabbatical from DH.

Anna Coleman is a Research Fellow and has worked at the National Primary Care Research and Development Centre (NPCRDC) since 2000. Prior to this she worked in various policy and research roles within local government. During 2006 she completed her PhD whilst investigating the development of Local Authority health scrutiny. Other current interests include partnership working, the development of practice based commissioning, health policy more generally and consultation with the public.

Mark Exworthy is Reader in Public Management and Policy in the School of Management at Royal Holloway-University of London. His research interests focus on decentralisation, professional-managerial relations and policy implementation, in relation to health-care. He has particular interests in policy responses to health inequalities.

Ian Greener is Senior Lecturer in Public Policy at Manchester Business School, as well as Director of Undergraduate Programmes. He is the author of a number of articles and book chapters on UK health policy including papers in Public Administration, Governance, Policy and Politics and Social Policy and Administration. He is particularly interested in how service users become positioned in particular roles by policy, and in the implications of this for service delivery. He lives in York, and has three children and a Pepsi Max habit to support.

Alison Hann is a tutor at the University of Wales Swansea. Her research interests focuses mainly on public health. She has published widely in the British White Cattle Society Journal.

Steve Harrison is Professor of Social Policy in the School of Social Sciences at the University of Manchester. He is currently on a long-term secondment to the National Primary Care Research and Development Centre. His research interests include health policy making, implementation and evaluation, and empirical research in health care organisations. He was formerly Professor of Health Policy and Politics at the University of Leeds, and has also worked in the civil service, the steel industry and the NHS. He tries to maintain another life as a folk musician.

Kathryn Jones is a Senior Research Fellow in the Health Policy Research Unit, Department of Public Policy, De Montfort University, Leicester. Her research interests include user involvement, patients' organisations, professional regulation and the pharmaceutical industry. Publications include *Speaking for Patients and Carers: Health Consumer Groups and the Policy Process* (with Rob Baggott and Judith Allsop, Palgrave Macmillan, 2005) and *Quality Assurance in Medical Regulation in an International Context* (with Judith Allsop, University of Lincoln, 2006). She has also published in *Sociology of Health and Illness*, *Health Expectations*, and *Policy and Politics*.

Ruth McDonald is Research Fellow at the National Primary Care Research and Development Centre, University of Manchester. Her research interests concern issues of change and resistance in organizations. Wherever possible she has explored these from inside the organization(s) concerned, examining amongst other things, the unintended consequences of change and its implications for individual identity. Recent research topics include the 'empowerment' of staff in a Primary Care Trust, threats to patient safety in the operating theatre and the new general medical practice (GP) contract. All of which is a far cry from her old job as an NHS finance director.

Chris Nottingham is Associate Dean for Research for the School of Law and Social Sciences and Reader in Contemporary History in Glasgow Caledonian University. His main current research interests are in Scottish health politics and the 'insecure professions' in health and welfare. He is currently working on a history of social work profession in Scotland from the 1960s to the present day, a documentary and oral history of the development of health education in Scotland, and editing a collection of studies of insecure professions. This year he is publishing an article on the development of the Dutch welfare system, (with Piet de Rooy of the University of Amsterdam) an article in *Medical History,* on medical social workers and social medicine in Scotland, and another article in the *International Review of Social History.* 'The Rise of the Insecure Professionals'.

Lucy O'Driscoll is a lecturer in the Faculty of Health at the University of East Anglia, in the UK. She was originally employed as a Lecturer in Physiotherapy, having worked as a Chartered Physiotherapist in the NHS for ten years. In her current post she teaches research skills to pre- and post-registration clinicians at Undergraduate and Masters levels. She is the Director for the Faculty's Post Graduate Taught Programmes and is the Course Director for the Faculty's Masters in Clinical Education. Her research focuses on health service policy, policy decision-making and policy implementation. This case study is drawn from works undertaken as part of her PhD.

Gillian Olumide teaches social science at the school of health science at Swansea University. Her main research interests are in the construction of racialised meanings in professional literatures and in the involvement of children in decision making about their health affairs. She has published in both these areas. Currently she is working on a piece of research to investigate the way race and ethnicity is taught through the Welsh nursing curriculum and is a member of the steering group of the Wales Ethnicity and Diversity in Health and Social Care Research Support Network (WEDHS).

Stephen Peckham is Senior Lecturer in Health Services Delivery and Organisation at the London School of Hygiene and Tropical Medicine. He worked in local government for a number of years before undertaking his degree and Masters courses. He was Head of Sociology and Social Policy at Oxford Brookes University from 1999 to 2005. His main research interests are in health policy analysis and is currently involved in research on inter-organisational aspects of performance and decentralised decision making in local health economies, changing workforce in out of hours care, patient choice and public health policy and ethics.

Calum Paton is Director of the Centre for Health Planning and Management at Keele University, where he is Professor of Health Policy. He is a political scientist who has recently published New Labour's State of Health: Political Economy, Public Policy and the NHS (Avebury, 2006). He has previously published many books on politics and on health policy. He is Editor-in-Chief of the International Journal of Health Planning and Management (Wiley.) From 2000 to 2006, he was Chair of the University Hospital of North Staffordshire NHS Trust.

Susan Pickard has degrees in Modern History and Social Anthropology and a PhD in Social Anthropology. Currently based at the National Primary Care Research and Development Centre, University of Manchester, she has researched and published in the areas of user involvement, accountability, contracts and marketing, ageing and old age and informal care-giving.

Martin Powell is Professor of Health and Social Policy at the Health Services Management Centre, University of Birmingham. He has research interests in the history of health policy, choice and consumerism, partnerships, equity and decentralisation. He is the author of 'Evaluating the NHS' (Open University Press, 1997) and editor of 'Understanding the Mixed Economy of Welfare' (Policy Press, 2007).

Acknowledgements

The Health Politics Group, (which is a specialist group supported by the Political Studies Association) has been in existence now for seventeen years, and has been convened by myself for the last twelve. The group has developed into a firm community of academic colleagues and friends who regularly attend the annual Oxford conferences, collaborate in research activities, publications and importantly, are a continuing source of support and encouragement to each other and to aspiring post graduates. The chapters in this volume are mainly drawn from papers given at the annual conferences in September 2005–6. Thanks are therefore due to the members of this group – not only those who have contributed to this volume, but to the many others who attend the conferences and offer their support, enthusiasm and ideas. Thanks must also go to the Political Studies Association who support the group with a yearly grant.

In addition, I would like to thank particular colleagues who have been especially supportive and helpful and deserve to be mentioned in dispatches, and these are Stephen Peckham, Professor Calum Paton, Chris Nottingham, Gillian Olumide, Roy Cunningham, Professor Rob Baggott and Ian Greener.

I would also like to thank Debbie Corothers, Peter Johnson, Sally Davey and Malcom Wiiliams at the West Wales Hospital Trust pharmacy for their friendship and support. And last but not least Roger Baker of Pentwyn Mwyn Computer Services for his help in preparing the typescript.

Acknowledgements

Introduction

Alison Hann

The politics of health have been characterised as emerging from a triangle of intersecting forces between the medical profession, civil society and the state (Salter, 2004), but this triangle of forces, though central, are not the only players on the field. Health policy is also heavily influenced by pressures from a variety of national and international sources as well as from inter-professional struggles and critiques. Added to this is, are the activities of non-governmental groups such as the media, the pharmaceutical industry, patient user groups, the 'empowered patient' to mention but a few, who are seeking to influence policy to reduce health inequalities, improve service provision, control costs and improve efficiency and effectiveness. The academic analysis of the relationship between politics and policy does not simply engage with the monitoring of changes in government policy, or indeed what happens in the NHS, important though this is. It has recently become increasingly interested in analysing the provision of health services within the NHS (and outside it) in terms of such things as social justice, equality and diversity, while also carefully scrutinising the political and ideological dimensions to health and health care.

This volume contributes to the ongoing critical analysis of policy making at two levels. Firstly at the 'macro' level of policy making at governmental level, and secondly at the intermediate level of professional institutional relationships and struggles, Following this general structure, we begin by looking at overarching influences on certain aspects of UK health policy. In the first chapter Nick Boyd examines the potential impact of the EU on the NHS in future years, and argues that this is growing for a number of reasons. It examines the policy drivers for this change, and these include legislative powers for the Union in public health; a greater acceptance that health care is one of the limbs of EU social policy; and the effects on health services of the efforts to complete the single market in Europe. There are also legal drivers for change coming from a series of European Court of Justice cases connected with patient mobility and the right of access to services provided in other EU countries. The chapter concludes by raising questions about how these developments impact on social insurance based systems as opposed to tax based systems, and sets out some thoughts for future developments, particularly in the light of EU enlargement. The second chapter, sharpens the focus to the political economy and politics of current health policy In England in order to unravel the underlying causes of problems in the NHS. Calum Paton begins with a focus on the complexities and contradictions facing any analysis of the politics of health policy. 2005–2006 saw the biggest 'crisis' in NHS funding, despite significant extra expenditure on the (English) NHS. The chapter disentangles the various forces, both on the 'supply side' and the 'demand side' and links the analysis to the 'four streams of policy' which are currently in tension with each other in the NHS. He starts with the perplexing question of how it is, that despite 'record investment' by New Labour, the deficit across NHS hospital Trusts and Primary Care Trusts (PCTs) in England for 2005–2006 was c. £1.2 billion. The 'cause', Paton concludes is due partly to poor statecraft and contradictory policies, and partly to poor service planning.

Chapter three, then moves on to look at one of the major planks of government health policy – that of decentralisation. However, the authors point out that it is possible to discern both centralist and decentralist movements at work in the UK. The chapter examines existing analytical frameworks of decentralisation in order to identify whether policy is decentralist or not and in doing so, identifies a number of problems that limit their value. Key problems, it seems, are related to the way decentralisation is conceptualised and defined. Existing frameworks tend to be also highly contextualised and are therefore of limited value when applied in different areas. They therefore propose a new framework which they suggest provides a more useful way of examining centralisation and decentralisation through a more sophisticated way of categorising policies and actions which avoids the problems suffered by other models.

The last chapter in this section examines the development of policy making in healthcare, and in order to gauge the extent to which policy making has been 'modernised' the author examines some specific examples of policy making. The M*odernising Government* White Paper (1999) set up the Governments programme for modernising policy making. The White Paper and the subsequent documents and initiatives that followed aimed to identify best practice policy making and disseminate it across Whitehall.

Six years later, has the goal been reached? To answer this question, this chapter will focus on the Department of Health (DOH) to assess whether the Department's policy making has improved. A standard best practice policy making will be used to benchmark two case studies of policy formulation – the drafting of the Mental Health Bill, and the reform of the generic medicines policy.

The overall conclusion is that progress on modernising policy making seriously and substantially has improved in many aspects. It is more inclusive than before, has improved cross-cutting work, the use of evidence and the quality of Regulatory Impact Assessments, etc. But, on the other hand, there are still signs of the prevalence of old practices and a hierarchical, closed and reactive policy making style. Effective joined up work is still missing. Also, there is a serious lack of thinking about implementation during the stages of policy formation. Policy makers are not straightforwardly identifiable and the lack of available data, reports and timely feedback to reflect accountability is still something to work on. The Department's style is still very reactive and there is a long way to go in using risk assessment techniques effectively.

The next section of the volume begins with two chapters which use Hirschman's framework to examine different aspects of health policy. The first, by Ian Greener, examines UK health policy documents to examine how 'choice' and 'responsiveness' are used to position both users and the public in particular roles in health services. It suggests that health consumerism is a process that has gradually appeared in the NHS through the gradual extension of the role afforded to patients with the goal of making health services more responsive. Utilising Hirschman's framework of exit, voice and loyalty I explore this relationship, suggesting that although there appears to be a strong causal link between choice and responsiveness in the documents, it does not necessarily work in the opposite direction. This is because our analysis of responsiveness suggests that there are other means of achieving this goal other than increasing choice through consumerist approaches to organisation.

The second, Susan Pickard uses the framework to analyse the interactions between users and health care. She examines the way in which Hirschman contrasts exit and voice as 'repercussion' mechanisms for making organisations responsive to users. However, the emergence of health-care quasi-markets and of network governance structures since Hirschman wrote necessitate revising his theory, for they complicate the relationship between government structures and recuperation mechanisms. Using a case study of nine Primary Care Trusts (PCTs) this chapter analyses the recuperation mechanisms, governance structures and relations between them in English primary care. User voice can be exercised through dedicated networks besides hierarchies. Besides the 'user exit' described by Hirschman, two new 'exit' mechanisms now exists in quasi-markets. Commissioner exit occurs when a third-party payer stops using a given provider. Professional proxy exit occurs when a General Practitioner (GP) fund holder (or analogous budget holder) behaves similarly. Neither exit mechanism requires the existence of mechanisms for user exit from healthcare purchasers, provided strong voice mechanisms exist instead to make commissioners responsive to users' demands. Establishing such voice mechanisms however is not straightforward, as the example of the English PCTs illustrates. In short, Pickard concludes that voice, the dominant mechanism for responding to users within the NHS is not working – perhaps other mechanisms may need to be strengthened (or weakened), though this, she admits is difficult due to the types of conflicting and contradictory accountability chains currently in place. Chapter seven by Harrison and MacDonald is also concerned with an examination of the interactions between the citizen and the policy making organisations within health care. Public consultation and user involvement in the decision making of public services can be related both to the debate about appropriate governance for individual services and to broader debates around democracy and citizenship in the UK. Although there is historically little evidence of such involvement having large impacts despite good intentions, the election of Labour in 1997 brought a greater emphasis on patient and public involvement (PPI) in the NHS. This was represented as a way of strengthening accountability to local communities, developing a health service that genuinely responds to patients and carers and promoting a sense of ownership and trust. Following the 2000 Local Government Act local government authorities have developed the role of overview and scrutiny, initially of their own internal functions, and since January 2003 extended to include local health services (health scrutiny). This is just one of a variety of related initiatives introduced to replace Community Health Councils (CHCs). The chapter examines the potential of health scrutiny and other related PPI initiatives for increasing the public voice in health related decision making. Research conducted by the National Primary Care Research and Development Centre around the implementation of health scrutiny between 2002 and 2005 is used to illustrate the analysis.

The next chapter by Harrison and Coleman is concerned with the way that the public are represented – until the reorganisation of the English National Health Service in 1974, the various institutions that administered it were also responsible for representing the public. Even though directly elected local government authorities provided only the public health and community services elements of the NHS, the appointed hospital management committees and executive councils for the family health services (general medical, dental and optical practitioners and pharmacists) had been assumed to be responsible both for managing the service and for representing the user and public interest. Indeed, some members of such authorities had chosen to take, though apparently rather ineffectively, a service user viewpoint (Levitt and Wall, 1984: 254). However, the area and regional health authorities created to run the newly-unified service from 1974 onwards were responsible only for its management (Levitt and Wall, 1984: 254), an arrangement that has survived the numerous subsequent reorganisations of these institutions. Since that time, the public representation function has been carried out by separate bodies, Community Health Councils (CHCs) from 1974 until their abolition in 2003, and since then by local government authorities exercising their responsibility for 'overview and scrutiny' of the NHS. The chapter compares these two regimes of representation in terms of their operation, origins and impact.

Chris Nottingham's chapter moves the debate into a new area – that of the interactions between the health professionals and health policy – in this instance, health promotion and public health, with particular reference to Scotland. He points out that there is currently a great deal of enthusiasm for public health policies among policy makers in the Health Services of the UK. The 'New Public Health' with its emphasis on health promotion and disease prevention has come of age. In Scotland in particular public health initiatives have been embraced with great enthusiasm. The appointment of Harry Burns, previously Director of Public Health for the Greater Glasgow Board of Health and much associated with campaigns against health inequalities, as Chief Medical Officer, sends a clear signal about how the direction of policy, as did the announcement of a ban on smoking in public places. In recent white papers it has been made clear that health professionals will be expected to take an active role in a 'health promoting service'. There is an explicit determination to tackle the legacy of poor health which is one of the more unfortunate aspects of Scotland's heritage.

The chapter raises a number of issues which might suggest that enthusiasm should be tempered with caution. Firstly, it is important to recognise that the academic literature does not agree as to the desirability and efficacy of such policies. Alongside those who are enthusiastic there are those who see such policies as an attempt by governments to extend their powers into areas which they should steer clear of. Social libertarians and 'Foucauldians' alike have warned of authoritarian strains in the 'New Public Health'. The author draws on recent research he has been involved in which throws light on this controversy. An historical examination of the rise and fall of medical social work in Scotland and a contemporary study of the activities of Health Visitors in health promotion in Glasgow to suggest that the active promotion of a 'social model' of health raises more complex issues than is often appreciated. Health professionals are for the most part well respected by their clients and the public in general. This owes something to the fact that they are seen as responding to health needs as experienced by the patients. However this authority could be weakened if they came to be seen as operating to an externally imposed agenda.

In Chapter ten, Lucy O'Driscoll moves into an analysis of a particular case of problem solving, by using the model of policy networks developed by Marsh & Smith. In particular she draws on the suggestion that the nature of policy networks may influence policy outcomes. Her chapter examines this idea through the analysis of an empirical case study, using policy network theory. The case study is one in which local NHS managers and clinicians collaborated to develop and implement a solution for protracted patient waiting for orthopaedic services in their Trust.

The chapter outlines the dimensions and importance of the policy problem locally and nationally, and explains the importance of examining the policy processes involved in managing patient waiting. The study Trust was analysed using the Rhodes and Marsh policy network typology. The chapter concludes by describing the structure and agency factors which were seen as key in influencing policy outcomes. It will also suggest that a new type of policy network, described as 'surrogate policy community' could be seen in this case. She suggests that such 'surrogate policy communities' may be seen at work wherever policy communities seek to share decision making with key stake holders, such as clinicians and hospital managers. She also considers the consequences of permitting decision-making to be undertaken by such a policy community.

The chapter by Gill Olumide considers a different kind of 'problem' solving. She examines not just the 'solution', but also, importantly, the way in which the 'problem' has been conceptualised by various commentators and policy makers. The focus of her chapter is the recent political desire to tackle diversity – however that might be understood. She examines the current fascination with the notion of diversity and the move away from policies and struggles which promote equality of opportunity in areas such as gender and disability to a view which embraces an 'umbrella' handling of inequality issues in public policy.

The question appears to demand an analysis not simply of how 'diversity' may be promoted but of why differently perceived differences have led to such a striking and persistent inequalities in the first place. Whether perceptions of, for example race or disability can be subsumed under a single diversity umbrella is a moot point. Without reference to the conditions of the emergence of social inequality, and perhaps more importantly to groups which enjoy a consistently share of social resources diversity oriented policy is bereft of foundation.

With particular reference to the UK NHS diversity policies and to the move to collapse existing inequalities quangoes into a single (state funded) equalities body the chapter aims to open up debate and to examine some of the common policy assumptions about differences in opportunity and outcome.

This is followed by another 'case study' of sorts, but from a totally different perspective. In this case, the practice of population immunisation is examined from the ethical perspective. It seeks to explore the relationship between evidence, ethics and public health policy, with particular reference to vaccination policy. There is a huge investment in vaccination programmes in the UK as a preventative public health measure to improve population health. However, vaccination remains a controversial issue and the subject of media and political debate, such as the furore around MMR demonstrates. The government and public health medicine justify the programmes as being both medically and ethically good as the evidence supporting population vaccination is strong and the benefits far outweigh the potential harm. This chapter questions the ethical and evidential basis of vaccination policy by examining whether the intervention does what it says it is supposed to do, whether there is good evidence to support it (including a discussion of what exactly constitutes evidence), the harms as well as the benefits caused by the intervention, and as a result, whether or not a population based vaccination policy is ethical. The interesting questions which link the previous two chapters is that they all question what is generally taken as being a self evident good nd subject them to a critical gaze. This could also be said of the chapter by Kathryn Jones who takes an unusual angle on the role of the pharmatceutical industry. In particular she explores the policies of the pharmaceutical industry in the UK. Drawing on interviews with representatives from the pharmaceutical industry, civil service and health consumer groups she examines the role of the pharmaceutical industry in the policy process. In particular, she explores issues relating to the regulation of the drugs industry, the drugs approval process and the growing links between health consumer groups and the pharmaceutical industry. This is especially timely given the recent Health Select Committee's (2005) report into the influence of the pharmaceutical industry.

The final chapter examines the impact of the new GMS (nGMS) contract within the changing organisational and policy context of the English NHS. It begins with outlining the current policy context for the English NHS before moving on to examine the current contractual arrangements for general practice. The next section then discusses the potential impacts on general practice in the UK. The chapter ends by discussing what some of the wider implications of the new contract might be in the UK more generally – particularly within the context of the development of differing health systems in Northern Ireland, Scotland and Wales.

This scope of this volume is therefore very wide. Together, each of the chapters offers a critical insight into the way in which health policy is formulated at almost every level, but it does not stop there. There is close attention to the ways in which ideologies, values, economics, micro-politics and even political expediency underpin the development of policy, the process of policy making and the way in which it is implemented or changed. These complexities are not 'dodged' by any of the contributors to this volume. This however, does not necessarily answer all the important questions raised – indeed one might argue that this is not the 'job' of the academic. Instead, what we aim to do is to pose questions?

References

Marsh, D., Smith, M.J. (2000) Understanding Policy Networks: towards a Dialectical Approach. *Political Studies*, **48**, 4–21.

Rhodes, R., Marsh, D. (1992) *Policy Networks in British Politics: A Critique of Existing Approaches*, in Marsh, D., and Rhodes, R. (eds) 'Policy Networks in British Government.' Clarendon Press: Oxford. pp. 1–26.

Rhodes, RAW. (1997) *Understanding Governance: Policy Networks, Governance, Reflexivity and Accountability.* Open University Press: Maidenhead, Berkshire.

Salter, B. (2004) *The New Politics of Medicine*, Palgrave Macmillan, Basingstoke.

Chapter 1

The Impact of the European Union on the NHS[1]

Nick Boyd

This chapter examines, from a UK Government perspective, the impact of developments in the European Union on the UK health service (the NHS). It examines UK Government policy to date on the role of the EU in health services and how various drivers in recent years have influenced and refined that policy position.

Existing UK Policy

The Labour administration which came to power in 1997 was committed to signing the social chapter of the European Treaty, and participating fully in the debates on social developments in Europe. As far as health services were concerned, however, it reconfirmed the position held by previous administrations that the organisation and delivery of health services was a member state responsibility: the Union had no competence to intervene in this area. During negotiations on the Amsterdam Treaty of 1998, the UK backed a specific reference in Article 152 of the new Treaty – in the public health chapter – which read:

> Community action in the field of public health shall fully respect the responsibilities of the Member States for the organisation and delivery of health services and medical care.

At the same time, the Government acknowledged that, while responsibility for the organisation and delivery of health care services needed to be retained at national level, there were some *public health* issues on which action at European level was needed in order to protect and improve the health of citizens of its Member States. Indeed, there were already powers in the Treaty of Maastricht for the Union to take supportive measures in the field of public health – which led to the public health programmes of the 1990s – and the Government also supported Commission initiatives to use single market powers in certain areas, such as tobacco control, to take legislative measures.

1 Presentation to a colloquium of the Politics of Health Group, Merton College, Oxford, 9 September 2005.

Drivers for Change

The years that followed implementation of the Amsterdam Treaty saw several drivers which affected this policy position.

The *strengthening of public health powers* in the Treaty raised questions about the grey area between 'public health measures' where the Union had new legislative powers – for example on the safety of blood, tissues and cells – and 'health service interventions' where it had no competence. In other words, it had competence to legislate on standards of safety in the procurement and transport of blood, but not on how it was used in clinical interventions.

Proposals for the new Constitutional Treaty (*proposed Article 179(4)(d)*) would have further strengthened these public health powers – particularly in the area of communicable disease prevention and control – no doubt giving rise to similar questions.

Discussions on *social protection* in the EU have developed in new directions, too. Whereas in earlier years, their focus had been on labour market policies and employment protection, they came to embrace pensions policy and social exclusion, too. The European Council decided to add to these three existing arms of social protection work the need for sustainable, accessible and quality health services. Since 2001-2 this latter field has been subjected to the 'Open Method of Coordination' process – a structured system of discussion between Commission and Member States to exchange best practice, and in some cases set objectives and carry out peer review and benchmarking.

Perhaps the most powerful driver for policy change has been the further *development of the single market* and the application of its rules to health service. It has always been the case that health services in Member States are directly influenced in one way or another by EU legislation, much of it based on internal market provisions in the Treaties. Since the 1970s there has for example been legislation to regulate licensing procedures for pharmaceutical products and, to a lesser extent, medical devices; and legislation on the mutual recognition of professional qualifications, including for doctors and nurses. Health and Safety provisions apply to the NHS workforce as to any other (e.g. the Working Time Directive). Similarly, the NHS must observe EU Directives on procurement.

However, from 1999 onwards there have been a series of highly influential decisions from the European Court of Justice establishing caselaw which applies internal market rules to the provision of, and access to, health services. These cases (e.g. Kohll and Dekker (1998); Smit-Geraets and Peerbooms (2001); Müller-Fauré and van Riet (2003) and others) arose often from referrals from Courts in member states considering complaints from individuals about the refusal of their sickness fund to reimburse treatment they had, without prior authorisation from their fund, sought in another EU member state. In some cases this was because the individual concerned could not access the treatment they wanted at home without waiting; in others, because the treatment was not available in their home country, or they found it more convenient to have it abroad.

Through these cases, the Court established several important principles. Some of the key ones were:

- EU single market rules do apply to health services, whether publicly or privately provided;
- The requirement for prior authorisation by a funder of health services to treatment abroad is an obstacle to the free movement of services, and thus in conflict with single market rules;
- There are however legitimate considerations to bear in mind when applying single market rules to health services – for example the need for Member States to plan hospital provision and to run their own social security systems: they can legitimately refuse to take action which would make such planning impossible or undermine the financial stability of their health system;
- A requirement for an individual to seek prior authorisation before going abroad for hospital treatment can be justified, but authorisation can only be refused in certain conditions. These include that the treatment in question is not part of the home member state's package; and that it can be provided in the home member state 'without undue delay'. There are others.

Although these cases all arose in the context of countries with social insurance systems, the ECJ confirmed in its decision on a case relating to the UK NHS (Mrs Watts) in 2006 that its caselaw applies to tax-based systems such as the NHS as well.

The significance of this caselaw is that it establishes that the Commission does have competence to propose measures, based on internal market provisions in the Treaty, concerned with ensuring freedom to provide health services across the EU, and the conditions under which European citizens can gain access to those services. In its original proposals in 2004 for a general Services Directive, the Commission did in fact include provisions relating to provision of and access to health services. The Council and the European Parliament did not believe that a general Directive applying to a wide range of services was an appropriate vehicle for dealing with sensitive and complex health service issues, and this part of the Directive was dropped. However, the Commission subsequently announced plans for separate health service-specific legislation, and their proposals for such legislation is expected in 2007. This is likely to cover the kinds of issues raised by the caselaw of the ECJ.

Enlargement

It is still too early to assess the full impact of the enlargement of the EU in 2004, but it is likely that this, too, will bring new perspectives regarding the role of the EU in health service policy. The 10 new member states represented the single largest expansion the EU had experienced, and created a new dynamic. The wealth gap between poorest and richest States was widened. The proportion of small to large Member States also grew significantly. In the original EU 15 there were 4 countries with a population of less than 6 million. In EU 25 there are 11. Many of these countries have relatively underdeveloped health service infrastructures, and also relatively weak health Ministries within Government. It is possible that they will look more actively to the Commission, and to the EU for support in capacity building in health services (for example on health technology assessment). Although they will be careful to safeguard their own policy control and guard against cost pressures arising from European actions, they may not have the same cautious attitude to EU active involvement in health service policy as some of the older Member States have traditionally had.

Conclusion

Taken together, these developments have created a new and different context for Member States to develop their thinking on the role of the EU in health services policy. There remains widespread acknowledgement in the Institutions of the EU that Member States are responsible for the organisation and delivery of health services, but the debate about how this responsibility relates to competences the EU has in the internal market and other areas is one in which all parties are now fully engaged.

Chapter 2

The Politics of NHS Deficits and NHS Re-form

Calum Paton

The perplexing question about the (English) NHS at the end of 2006, which would strike the proverbial 'Man from Mars', is how it has seen what New Labour likes to call 'record investment' (actually expenditure, as investment is mostly private) yet a major structural problem with record deficits. This question is indeed perplexing not only to a putative Man from Mars but also to the Prime Minister and New Labour Health Ministers; to senior managers and clinicians; and (of course) to the long-suffering, much spun-upon NHS staff and English public. For the scale of the deficit as Financial Year 2005–2006 progressed was a major surprise on an increasing scale as it was reported 'up the line' from individual Trusts, to Strategic Health Authorities, to the Department of Health management team, to health Ministers and finally to the Prime Minister.

The deficit across NHS hospital Trusts and Primary Care Trusts (PCTs) in England for 2005–2006 was c. £1.2 billion (although the government in the end artificially reduced the figure to c. £550,000 by 'raiding' education, training, public health and mental health budgets – thus committing the cardinal sin of 'brokerage to hide deficits' for which it was simultaneously berating the NHS). The reason it was a surprise of increasing size as the news was reported 'up the line' was primarily because of the cultural politics of the NHS.

A Very British (Pre-) Stalinism

This culture can be summed up in the memorable phrase from across the Atlantic, 'kiss up, kick down.' NHS Trust bosses are nervous of reporting deficits and seek to under-report until it's too late. Apparatchiks at Strategic Health Authorities (SHAs), primarily Chairs, Chief Executives and Directors of Finance, do what apparatchiks do – seek to please their superiors in the short term and shift blame 'down the line' in the longer line when the former (lack of) strategy unravels. For example, in the Shropshire and Staffordshire Health Authority, half-way through the financial year, the SHA was reporting 'break-even'. In the end, the SHA-wide deficit was c. £60 million.

The NHS Chief Executive and his management team at the Department of Health are nervous of Ministers such as Alan Milburn (Health Secretary from 1999 to 2003) and John Reid (Health Secretary from 2003 to 2005) with a reputation for what we might call the robust approach - and so fail to tell the Emperor that he has no clothes, or that at least his clothes are looking threadbare. This left the successor Secretary of State who inherited the problem, Patricia Hewitt, open to ridicule when the tactic of denial (of deficits and pending knee-jerk job cuts proposed by 'macho managers' seeking to use crisis to 'kiss up') was undermined by the facts unravelling in the media (which cannot be blamed, in this case, for reporting reality). From *The Guardian* to *The Daily Telegraph*, she was accused (respectively) of scapegoating (Paton, 2006a) and of sailing through the NHS's 'Potemkin hospitals' (*Daily Telegraph*, 2006) like Catherine the Great viewing the facades of idyllic riverbank villages, oblivious to the truth behind the facades assembled by apparatchiks.

The time-dishonoured tactic of Ministerial head-in-the-sand applied: first, deny that the problem exists; then deny the problem is a large one; then assert that, where deficits are large, they are purely local and caused by bad local management; then, when this unravels, claim that Ministers were not apprised of the real situation (hence one of the reasons for the 'resignation' of the NHS Chief Executive and Department of Health Permanent Secretary Sir Nigel Crisp in March 2006, as the end of the financial year loomed); then – when, on reflection, Ministerial ignorance would (rightly) seem incompetent – claim that 2005-6 was a 'one-off' and indeed a consequence of the government's reform programme 'flushing out' historical problems. Well, up to a point, Lord Copper. The problem for the government was that the 'historical problems' were of recent vintage, and largely down to New Labour's amateurish zeal in policy-making causing financial anarchy in the English NHS.

Quis Custodes Custodiet?

So how did a creditable record on NHS expenditure after 2002, following the recommendations of the Chancellor's appointed advisor, Derek Wanless, come to co-exist with record deficits? It is fair to say that the analysis carried out so far has been incomplete. Independent but 'insider' commentators such as the (statutory) Audit Commission and the (non-statutory) King's Fund, parliamentary inquiries such as that by the Health Select Committee of the House of Commons (2006) and pro-market think-tanks such as Reform have emphasised (respectively) technical factors, short-term factors and ideologically-rooted explanations.

Of the above, the King's Fund published easily the best explanation for the deficit crisis (Palmer, 2006), but Palmer's paper sought the solution in 'strategic commissioning', more technically competent tariffs for paying providers and clearer system regulation. Of these, the first was the old, old story (see below) and the third presents a 'rational' case for better regulation and/or management of the market which is unimpeachable on its own terms but exclusive of the main political dynamic of the NHS – a 'garbage can' approach to policy initiatives (Paton, 2006).

The Audit Commission bars itself from political analysis (and in any case builds its national analysis from local investigations – regular annual audits and Public Interest Reports - by accountants whose technical skills are generally in inverse proportion to their understanding of the budgetary politics of the NHS). The

King's Fund's analysis, as just suggested, might be described as 'necessary but not sufficient' – good as far as it goes. The Commons Select Committee, in 2006, has borne the hallmark of many such committees – enough government quasi-loyalists (the disappointed and the dispossessed, from New Labour's ranks, yes, but not out-and-out rebels) to tone down radical criticism of the Executive, with awareness of electoral politics leading to an eschewal of comments which could form (in this case) Tory soundbites.

Think-tanks such as Reform and Civitas (incorporating the Institute of Economic Affairs' former Health Unit) have sought the answer in privatisation (of one sort or another) irrespective of the question. They have seen deficits as a problem of public sector productivity per se i.e. the fault of the public sector rather than of political initiatives foisted on the public sector which create contradictory objectives and lower productivity.

Inadequate Policy Levers . . . or Contradictory Policies

The conventional analysis refers euphemistically to 'inadequate policy levers' (Palmer, 2006). This holds out the prospect of all good men and true refining the system in response to evidence. Instead, I would argue that it is contradictory policies which are at fault, and that they have their origin in the politics (Paton, 2006). Furthermore, even assuming a quasi-rational policy process, there is no evidence that 'improved commissioning' within a market NHS, as opposed to proper service planning, will get round the problems. I explore the former point now, and the latter point later in this chapter.

Let us consider tacit policy contradictions in as concrete a way as possible. For example, targets may be worthwhile in principle (or in moderation) but expensive at the margin. A classic example was the '98 per cent A and E target', mandating that 98 per cent of patients who arrive at Accident and Emergency in hospitals must be admitted, treated or discharged within four hours of arrival (or four and one-quarter hours of the ambulance arriving at the hospital i.e. the 'clock starts' soon after the ambulance arrival whether or not the patient stays in the ambulance while awaiting admission or not ... to prevent the perverse incentive of 'ambulance blocking' to prevent the clock being started ... Such was the NHS in 2005–2006!)

Subjectively, the target per se was good – it focussed the managerial mind wonderfully upon the type of wait which is genuinely distressing to patients and families. Yet 'ratcheting it up' from 94 per cent to 98 per cent (one of Health Secretary Alan Milburn's last gifts to the NHS) meant that a lot of money had to be spent in many Trusts 'at the margin' (preventing relatively few 'breaches' of the target) which could have been spent to much greater effect in terms of overall hospital 'productivity.'

Now if politicians want to say, 'we want to diminish overall productivity in order to pursue a hallowed objective', then let them – there is nothing incoherent about that, and it is even more politically acceptable if they are accountable in some way for the decision. (It's what Prime Minister Blair might call a 'hard choice!') But of course they do not say that. They indicate, with the left hand, that all targets must be met, and with the right hand that productivity is to be maximised.

The reality in 2005–2006 was that some government policies and targets directly lowered hospital productivity. Pay settlements and 'reforms' did so, as did the other 'four Ps' (see below). Additionally however, targets themselves lowered aggregate productivity further – and differentially across the hospital sector, depending upon local needs, resources, historic capacity and local 'demand management' (e.g. how well PCTs kept patients away from A and E by managing (e.g.) chronic conditions in the community ... or not.)

The-then Chief Executive of the NHS Nigel Crisp rightly argued that investing in staff (recruitment, retention and re-training in a global economy, one might put it) should be a matter for praise not blame. But, as ever, Ministers did not attempt to quantify the timeframe within which there would be 'payback' through increased productivity (or indeed the costs of employing more, more productive staff in terms of the need to pay for more aggregate output from the NHS). It is not rocket science that in the short term there would be 'lower productivity'. But by running scared from a mature debate, the government ran scared from the stridency of the right-wing think-tanks as well as from the 'official stats' which screamed 'lower hospital productivity', egged on by the media and by no means only the tabloids.

None of the analyses from such sources have sought a political root cause for deficits – or situated them in unstable local health economies rather than individual Trusts. They have missed the wood in assiduously classifying various trees. This chapter contends that we must look to the contradictory and clashing policy initiatives and neurotically-frequent structural re-organisations promoted by New Labour from 1997, and especially after 2002. It was then that Blair's conversion to a supra-Thatcherite view of public service reform (and later his quest for a legacy) led to the Walt Disney's Fantasia's Sorcerer's Apprentice approach to policy: little brushes rush in all directions in earnest endeavour – well-intentioned yet flooding the house under the ineffectual supervision of Mickey Mouse.

The Blairite 'Sofa' Policy Process

For make no mistake: health policy (for England) has not only been amateurish in the extreme but also has been made directly from the office of the Prime Minister (Meyer, 2005; Butler, 2005) especially after his trusted acolyte and New Labour 'outrider' Alan Milburn vacated Richmond House (the Whitehall home of the Department of Health). Prime Ministerial health advisers, such as Simon Stevens, Julian le Grand and Paul Corrigan, have been the policy champions for health reform, in some cases (Stevens and Corrigan) providing a bridge to the Department of Health given their origin as political advisers to Health Secretaries.

The Department of Health (DoH) has been follower, not leader, in health policy – reflecting the centralist nature of the Blair Executive. Independent advice to Ministers in the DoH from career civil servants, already waning due to the relative marginalisation of the Permanent Secretary (PS) following the Griffiths reforms of 1983, was diminished further by unifying the roles of Permanent Secretary to the

DoH and Chief Executive (CE) of the NHS, in Autumn 2000 when Nigel Crisp was appointed. In effect both roles were now filled by political appointments.

With the re-separation of the roles in summer 2006 (with Hugh Taylor Acting PS and career NHS manager David Nicholson as the new CE), both separate appointments are still de facto political. The CE, for example, while from the 'chessboard' style of management, with a record of seeking results by moving pieces on the board in a dirigiste manner - and also (more overtly) a believer in planned reconfigurations of health services – is not in a position to give Sir Humphrey-style lectures to Ministers (a la Yes Minister). Sir Humphrey had his faults – arrogance and scepticism about politicians' priorities – but his 'new public management' alter ego is structurally committed to 'kiss up, kick down.'

This essay thus puts the technical and piecemeal explanations for deficit in political context – acknowledging some of the conventional explanations (such as uncosted pay initiatives, the costs of Private Finance Initiatives et al.) but locating them in a wider framework.

The Causes of Deficit – The Four 'P's . . . and the 'T' word

The four 'P's are: policies in conflict; purchasing by PCTs creating anarchy; privatisation (through both the Private Finance Initiative for capital and the 'top-slicing' of revenue budgets to pump-prime the private sector with a generosity which would have amazed even Mrs. Thatcher); and pay reform, which was ill thought out and poorly costed. Within these overall categories, particular factors loomed large in different parts of the NHS across England. For example, the new policy of Payment by Results hit certain specialist services hard through no fault of their own but through the new formula for reimbursement being faulty (Palmer, 2006).

In the dry language of economics, there were both 'supply' and 'demand' factors to explain deficits – with different effects in different locations. 'Technical' words such as supply and demand may have political and structural explanations behind them, however. For example, hospital 'supply' and productivity may be retarded by the perverse behaviour of NHS purchasers (PCTs) misleadingly called commissioners, when even purchasing was beyond most of them - and not (just) by internal management within hospitals. Such behaviour, in turn may be encouraged by perverse incentives set up by the 'policy structure' (i.e. clashing national policies and initiatives whose effect 'on the ground' is known little and cared-about less by Ministers and the 'policy wonks' who advise them.)

Additionally to the four 'P's (which contain both demand and supply factors) one can add the 'T' word – targets (see above). Especially before the 2005 general election, the word on the NHS street, promulgated from above, was 'meeting the targets'. Some of the targets were actually rather good, and a helpful catalyst to taking patients' concerns seriously. Some were less so; the overall combination was a rag-bag. Neither the 'good' nor the 'bad' aspect of targets is the point here, however. The pre-election target regime said (off the record), 'meet the targets and worry about the money later (no job cuts in election year, please)'. For hospitals in poor areas (with an imbalance of need and local resources, especially where the

PCTs did not have in-year budgets which recognised that need and especially where the PCT configuration was wasteful), this might mean huge pressure.

At the very least it would require PCTs to work hand-in-glove with hospitals to ensure that they were seeking the same level of success with the same targets. Yet this was often absent. The 'policy strand' of collaboration was usually marginalised by a sectarianism encouraged by: separate targets for PCTs and hospitals (such that the former did not care if the latter failed theirs); the 'purchaser/provider split' inherited from the Conservatives and deepened by Alan Milburn's dysfunctional reform of 2001, Shifting the Balance of Power (DoH, 2001); and the 'new market' after 2002, which provided new disincentives to collaboration. Hospitals might thus end up between a rock and a hard place in seeking to meet ambitious targets and also break even financially.

Of Good and Bad Trusts

Some deficits, of course, could be due to 'bad internal management' in the Trust, but these were probably a minority. A notorious minority, to be sure: much later, in late 2006, Secretary Hewitt was right to point to the NHS financial regime 'making her hair stand on end' (2006) (albeit a curious claim by one of the in-house stalwarts of New Labour after nearly ten years of New Labour stewardship of the NHS!) The problem was that she was making the right generalisation based on the wrong examples, and therefore learning the wrong lessons.

In the early 2000s, some of the best-managed hospitals both broke even and met (most) targets. By the time StBoP and other initiatives had done their worst, roughly by 2004 to 2006, this was no longer sustainable *if* other aspects of the 'four Ps' were also hitting hard. As a result, some notably well-managed hospitals went into deficit just at the time that the government was panicking about the national deficit; and the examples chosen by Hewitt and her team to illustrate bad management, labyrinthine financial regimes or both were not the right ones.

In a nutshell, some hospitals in deficit were poorly-managed, some were not; some breaking even were well-managed and lucky, some were badly-managed and luckier-still (in terms of which of the 'four P' and other factors hit in-year). Yet in explaining deficits, the Audit Commission (AC) (2006) sought refuge in a narrow range of technicalia about the processes of budget-setting, on the one hand, and bland homilies about the nature of Boards, on the other.

The trouble was that the former ignored the politics of the budgetary process: if PCTs were cutting the budget yet failing to manage demand, was a hospital supposed to take the PCT's word even when the evidence belied it, or set an appropriate budget given unavoidable workload? Regarding the latter: when Boards began to display dysfunctional behaviour, was this the cause if a slide into deficit or a reaction to…? Clearly it could be either or both. Yet the AC report was based on local Audit Commission work (i.e. by District Audit), which eschewed subtle or even basic political-structural factors in 'explaining' deficits.

The Prime Minister, Tony Blair, was keen to argue from the 'no pain, no gain' perspective: that large deficits were due to his hallowed 'public sector reforms' flushing out poor performers. The problem was that the high noon for deficits (one hopes it was…!) had come in 2005–2006, the year before his (and they were his, or rather his advisers') most recent NHS reforms began to be implemented!

These reforms would – in theory – ensure that Payment by Results allowed hospitals to be paid for the work they did … at tariff per case and not above, to be sure, but at least paid for the actual volume of work with which the hospital was confronted. It was exactly the absence of proper payment for volume (for NHS Trusts which had not become more 'independent' Foundation Trusts, and so could not seek legal redress for under-payment) which had driven some well-managed Trusts into deficit. The fact that Foundation Trusts (FTs) have a better financial record in 2005–2006 is a rather puerile truism rather than a testimony to a brave new world: quite simply, these Trusts can enforce payment for work done (and mostly have), whereas NHS hospital Trusts cannot. At best they will seek adjudication or arbitration from SHAs in their disputes with PCTs.

The politics of this process in 2005–2006 must be examined if we are to understand the scapegoating of (mostly) hospitals. SHA apparatchiks wish to concentrate deficits in as few organisations as possible, so they can be 'managed.' Politicians wish the same – to give spurious plausibility to their claim that deficits are down to a few individual organisations. (A memorable soundbite, or rather mantra endlessly repeated, from junior health Ministers to PM and Chancellor, from January to September 2006, was that '50 per cent of the deficit was in 6 (then 7, then 8, then 9!) per cent Trusts'. If we pause, we can see that this is meaningless – what about the other 50 per cent? – even before we explore how many organisations really share the deficit. For example, in North Staffordshire, the hospital was 'dumped' with most of the deficit (two-thirds of which was unpaid bills by the PCTs – bad debt rather than bad management) yet most agencies, including all the PCTs, were much more in deficit than official returns suggested.

Poorly-managed Trusts which had been concealing deficits for years through 'bungs' or brokerage from Regions (before 2002) and SHAs (after 2002) were the real examples of the labyrinthine financial regime which made Hewitt's hair stand on end, and which she now wanted the Chairman of the Audit Commission to investigate. But they were old news at the local and regional levels, and not on the radar screen at the national level when the national crisis hit. The technical examination of the *new* deficits by statutory reviewers and inspectors (such as Audit) combined with Ministers' desires to 'explain away' deficits as caused by a 'few bad apples' rather than wider systemic faults to produce a focus upon individual Trusts rather than wider 'health economies'.

Healthcare Standards and Resources

The NHS financial regime did need improvement. Under the old 'star system'; up to 2005, it was possible to 'cover up' deficits through arranged brokerage. Ironically the Trust I chaired (University Hospital of North Staffordshire) never needed such up to 2005; and the then Chief Executive and I lobbied the HCC (Healthcare Commission) in 2004 for a more accurate assessment of finances than provided under the star system.

The new 'standards'-based system (HealthCare Commission, 2006) does this, in part. Unfortunately it is a 'good system in the wrong circumstances'. Trusts rated as 'weak' or 'fair' in finance many be badly managed'; or they may be adversely affected by local provider and commissioner configurations and behaviour; national policy or all of these. Which factors come into play depend upon things like presence or absence of PFI; presence or absence of significant 'top-slicing' to Independent Sector Treatment Centres; the local effects of PBR; pay settlements et al.

Also, it is not true that 'generally Trusts do well or badly in both finance and quality' as Department of Health spin suggests. The HCC league tables published in October 2006 make that clear. In short; some do well in both; some spend to achieve targets and quality; some break even at the cost of quality; and some do badly in both!

Moreover, one has to get behind the data. For example, qualitative 'standards' (as opposed to quantitative 'targets') can be good; or they can be a fudge, in which self-assessment (only 'verified' by patient/public involvement or Local Authority Scrutiny) does not provide consistency in comparison from one area to another. The HCC only inspects by exception (now, unlike the much-maligned Commission for Health Improvement, its predecessor); and unlike in Scotland where NHS Quality Improvement Scotland assesses 'standards' but with national criteria for in-depth (through peer-review) working with Trusts.

In the new HCC financial standards, for example, some are 'hard/quantitative (e.g. 'no deficit') and some are 'soft/process' (e.g. 'Trust Board has an audit trail showing compliance with PCT contracting intentions'.) Yet the later may be assessed by 'tick box' as if the issue was purely technical, whereas confusions in national and local policy may make (for example) a PCTs 'contracting' intentions 'irrelevant to reality!'

In short, some of the 'data' may be fairly meaningless, if not misleading – or at least not a valid or fair basis for judgements about governance, financial or otherwise.

Of Deficits and Reform

Political strategy is often 'emergent' rather than 'rational'. Thus it was with the deficit story. Eventually (strictly behind closed doors) some Ministers began to see that all was not as it seemed; they came to see that they were in danger of believing the government's own rhetoric.

Many deficits had been caused, not by the 'new market' (in which hospitals were 'paid by results') but by the incoherent combination of policies up to 2005–2006 – principally Milburn's Shifting the Balance of Power, a 'devolution' which actually deepened the conflict between 'purchasers (commissioners) and providers', combined with centralist targets, on the one hand, and exhortations to local collaboration (against the grain!), on the other hand.

In a nutshell, purchasers passed the buck to providers, as in the Tories' market in the 1990s (Paton, 1998) Additionally, the conflict of interest for purchasers/ commissioners was now deepened and localised, as small PCTs feathered their own nests before seeing what they had left over to pay the hospital. At its worst, the NHS business model had become fantasy supermarkets – a squabbling and dysfunctional family (of local PCTs) rushes through the supermarket (hospital), grabbing goodies off the shelf, then charging past the cashier, throwing some coins and shouting over their shoulder, that's all we're prepared to 'commission!'

The problem was that, sorting this out would mean ensuring that hospitals were paid properly – according to the new 'tariff' created under the Payment by Results policy. Bluntly this was unaffordable. So the pertinent news from late 2006 regarding financial strategy is that reimbursement is to be reduced for cases above the levels which the (newly-reorganised) PCTs wish to commission. What this will do is two-fold – firstly, reintroduce price competition by the backdoor (cheaper providers will be able to manage better under this system), which was an overt 'no, no' for the new system of patient choice; and, secondly, squeeze hospitals overall.

The latter is therefore rationalised by the 'emergent strategy' of a radical shift to care outside the hospital, 'in the community'. Hence the White Paper, Our health, Our Care, Our Say (2006). When heroic assumptions were made in the early 1990s to a similar end, New Labour found it had to increase the hospital bed stock when it came to power. Now it is abruptly reversing that policy, and undermining its own planned (and needed) investment in hospitals.

Farcically, New Labour has now re-discovered what Labour knew in 1994 (and which David Cameron's Tories, rapidly shedding their baggage from Cameron's former boss Norman Lamont, the originator of the PFI, wish now to claim – that the Private Finance Initiative was very costly and fairly inflexible (McKee et al, 2006). So it has now unbundled the schemes 'in the pipeline' which it itself had promoted through the bureaucratic and time-consuming (of senior NHS leaders' time) process of approval by the Treasury's Capital Investment Branch and the DoH's Private Finance Unit.

Joined-up?

One of New Labour's buzz-words in the early days was 'joined up government' (for which read both policy-making and implementation.) The recent reiteration of the 'shift to the community' in the NHS provides an example of policy, and especially implementation, in its least joined-up guise (and by implementation I refer to coherence in strategy led by politicians, not something which can be blamed on 'managers' either on the bridge or in the bowels of the health service).

One of the NHS's recent 'turnaround managers' (Antony Sumara, at the end of 2006 leading financial 'turnaround' in London), is on record as describing the system as 'bizarre' (Select Committee on Health, 2006) whereby hospitals in deficit can be sacking nurses before the community services (which will provide alternative care) are geared up even to knowing, let alone employing, nurses as part of their strategy. In a nutshell, as well as a farcical failure jointly to plan services for the different sectors of hospital and community – a consequence of the market NHS with its atomised health providers and 'commissioners' (euphemism again!) – such skilled professionals may be lost to the English NHS , as they emigrate, or lost to the health sector, as they leave the health arena.

Department of Health 'chiefs' tend to blame local management and leadership for deficits, in an environment of course where blaming their political masters would be severely career-limiting! But even the government's appointed 'turnaround managers' – such as Antony Sumara – sometimes acknowledge the wider systemic factors (such as the diversion of funds to private treatment centres) (Select Committee, 2006). They often get back 'on message' by also blaming local leadership, especially of finance. Yet this may ignore the politics of the budgetary process (see above) and attribute system failure to individual Trusts. Besides it is pretty rich for 'here today, gone tomorrow' turnaround managers to blame 'leadership', which requires commitment on a long-term basis.

'Turnaround' of finances in the NHS moreover is subject to the 'double whammy' of the Treasury's Resource Accounting and Budgeting (RAB) methodology, which is a disastrous regime for hospitals, and for those operating in a market on particular (a deficit of £10 million means cuts of £30 million the following year) (Paton, 2006; Palmer, 2006); plans for hospital and community are often treated separately; and hospitals are frequently scapegoated in the manner described above in a marriage of convenience between Ministers and managers. The Audit Commission was asked in Spring 2006 by the Health Secretary to investigate the NHS financial regime, including the RAB methodology; and it recommended (later in 2006) that the RAB approach be suspended.

Of Policy Pies . . . Four (and Twenty) Stages of Reform

By the end of Financial Year 2005–2006, the Secretary of State was in her counting-house, counting out the money and pledging, 'never again ….'; that the NHS would break even in 2006–2007 and that she could be judged by that pledge. The current confused policy regime in the NHS can be seen to contain significant perverse incentives. What are the prospects that relying more on 'the market', and allegedly tougher financial regime, will make things better?

When New Labour came to power, their first 'reform' (actually, merely a tidying-up of the policy trends they inherited from the outgoing Tories) consisted in the rhetoric of collaboration (and the 'third way'), accompanied by the reality of Primary Care Groups (to become Trusts), which were the Tories' 'Total Purchasing Pilots' generalised (and reined in, to 'abolish the market'). The second phase of reform consisted in the 'new centralism', the high noon of Milburn's targets. The third era was the misleadingly-named 'devolution', 'Shifting the Balance of Power' (allegedly to the 'clinical frontline', but never less so in practice), and ushered in the structural causes of the deficits of 2005–2006. The fourth phase is the 'hard market reforms', which kick in in earnest in 2006–2007 (unless political compromise intervenes).

Let us look at the market per se and then at the prospects for the 'new regime' to restore financial balance to the NHS at both national and local levels.

Firstly, squeezing hospitals as a means of 'forcing' what are termed efficiencies but may simply be economies may well combine with the tariff regime (Payment by

Results) such that individual provider Trusts make individual decisions which lead to both omission and overlap in the overall NHS menu of services (Paton, 2007).

Secondly, using the RAB methodology may lock hospitals in deficit (Paton, 2007) (including efficient hospitals) into a vicious circle of decline.

Thirdly, competition between hospitals may be a zero-sum game, as patients 'choose' for their 'elective' procedures as a result of negative publicity yet without positive knowledge of the alternative.

This will apply particularly if (fourthly) NHS hospitals seek to avoid 'demanding consumers', knowing that (especially in the environment of deficits and therefore 'cuts') they cannot compete with the pump-primed private sector. They may therefore seek to specialise in these services (specialised and/or emergency) where they are local 'monopolies' and therefore can act as 'lazy monopolists' which allow costs to drift up as long as they break even and 'satisfice' rather than 'maximise' quality. Hirschman (1970) has analysed such 'lazy monopolists', against the conventional wisdom that monopolies always behave as market maximisers of profit.

Fifthly, if NHS Trusts do not compete as neo-classical theory suggests, then – as Hirschman again puts it – 'competition may comfort monopoly' (Paton, 2007).

Sixthly and crucially, the market may work too quickly – which will be especially disastrous if it is the 'wrong hospitals' which close (or contract, or decline in service-mix or quality or both.) The following section suggests that, in both of the main policy regimes since New Labour began to 'devolve and marketise' i.e. from 2002–to 2005/2006; and from 2006 onwards, both 'good and bad hospitals' may be caught in a deficit cycle which is outside their control. To some extent Primary Care Trusts (PCTs) are also constrained, but – as resource holders – they can 'simply turn off the tap' (albeit failing on strategic objectives and hurting others i.e. hospitals), rather than being forced into deficit.

This is the fundamental flaw of the 'purchaser (commissioner)/provider split': it creates a buck-passing culture, especially from payer to provider – as much in the NHS as in the privatised UK railways which separated track from trains (Jenkins, 2006).

Deficits . . . Two Stages

The pre-2006 deficits, as outlined above, have been caused by the 'four Ps', plus targets, plus more traditional factors such as under-resourced areas interacting with the more recent factors (for example, poor areas seeking to meet their targets against a backdrop of fragmented PCTs failing to come together to make, let alone implement, coherent strategic plans).

The first 'P' – pay – actually is complex, and the soundbite inevitably simplifies this complexity. Hospitals have faced the new consultant contract; PCTs the new GP contract; both, but especially hospitals, have faced the deepening 'bite' of the European Working Time Directive. Additionally, the 'cost of risk' has grown significantly (for example the Clinical Negligence Scheme for Trusts). Add to this the local costs of Connecting for Health, the major IM and T initiative.

Privatisation covers both demand and supply factors. Resources for NHS Trusts are reduced by the government's policy of not only encouraging but pump-priming (and often subsidising) the private sector of provision. On the supply side, the costs of the Private Finance Initiative have (differentially) hit (mostly hospital) Trusts in two ways – the cost of private capital; and the costs of 'dressing up the bride' i.e. of preparing the public estate for PFI (e.g. impairment costs).

The other two 'Ps': PCTs/purchasing and policy confusion – have briefly been set out above.

If we call this the first stage of deficits, what are the prospects that the 'new regime' after 2006 will change things – and will it be a new regime?

In a nutshell, there will still be a contradiction between choice and strategic planning (or what Palmer (op.cit.) calls, in more technical language, a tension between 'strategic purchasing' and the current form of Payment by Results (PbR)). There is not enough money in the system, despite the extra allocations up to 2007–2008, to reconfigure hospital services, build capacity in the community, and allow free choice (i.e. run enough excess capacity so that declining and new services and networks can co-exist with enough capacity both to allow patients to choose any provider and also allow PCTs to pay all these providers by workload.

There is a tension between the 'PbR' market and a market managed by what Palmer calls 'strategic commissioners' – who in fact turn out to be the purchasers of the 1990s, using price competition and a declining tariff for 'over-performance' (usually the poor old hospitals facing admissions which the PCT cannot control on their behalf).

Managing the transition to the market – as in the 1990s – has meant imperfect compromises. For example, transitional funding devices, such as the 'PPA' (Purchasing Parity Allocation), have been advocated to protect PCTs who face bigger bills as a result of PbR. Yet they have muddied the waters of needs-based allocations, as well as relying on 'purchaser/provider cooperation' to make the tariff work (i.e. make over-tariff services cheaper and yet also ensure that a key incentive in the system – for hospitals to maximise admissions *if* they are paid, and PCTs to minimise them – does not bankrupt the system along the way.

Overall, PCTs may be able to break even only by 'refusing to pay.' Thus, as now, hospitals which are well-managed may face real patient demand yet inadequate financial demand and excess capacity which the formulae (both for capital charging and for repayment of deficit) triple-count. Add to this a flawed PbR and a pot-pourri of the pre-2006 causes of deficit, and – to quote Ronald Reagan – 'you ain't seen nothin' yet'!

References

Audit Commission (2006), *NHS Deficits* (July), Audit Commission, London (see also Audit Commission Website on recommendations for financial reform).

Butler, R. (2006), *Iraq Inquiry*, TSO, London.

Daily Telegraph (5 April, 2006), 'Potemkin Hospitals'.

Department of Health (2001), *Shifting the Balance of Power*, Department of Health, London.

HealthCare Commission (2006), *NHS Standards*, HealthCare Commission, London.

Hewitt, P. (8 September, 2006), Interview with John Carvel, *Guardian*.

Hirschman, A. (1970), *Exit, Voice and Loyalty*, Harvard University Press, Cambridge, MA.

Jenkins, S. (2006), *Thatcher and Sons: A Revolution in Three Acts*, Allen Lane, London.

McKee, M. et al. (2006), *Public-Private Partnerships for Hospitals*, Bulletin of the World Health Organization, November, **84**(11).

Meyer, C. (2005), *DC Confidential*, Weidenfeld and Nicholson, London.

Palmer, K. (2006), *NHS Reform: Getting Back on Track*, Kings Fund, London.

Paton, C. et al. (1998), *Competition and Planning in the NHS: The Consequences of the Reforms* (2nd edn), Stanley Thornes, Cheltenham.

Paton, C. (2006), *New Labour's State of Health: Political Economy, Public Policy and the NHS*, Ashgate, Aldershot.

Paton, C. (22 September, 2006a), 'Patricia Hewitt is blaming my hospital for financial chaos which her party created', *Guardian*.

Paton, C (5 April, 2006b), 'Blair Reforms Wrecking the NHS', *Daily Telegraph*, p. 2.

Paton, C. (2007), 'Visible Hand or Invisible Fist? Choice in the English NHS', *Journal of Health Economics*, Policy and Law.

Select Committee on Health (2006), *NHS Deficits: Hearings*, House of Commons/TSO.

Select Committee on Health (2006/2007), *Final Report*, TSO.

Chapter 3

Analysing Health Services Decentralisation in the UK

Stephen Peckham, Mark Exworthy, Martin Powell and Ian Greener

The organisational history of the health service is one that has seen the balance between centralisation and decentralisation in a state of constant flux (Klein, 2001; Klein, 2003). The emphasis on a more decentralist approach, "new localism", is a central pillar of the government's strategy across a number of sectors including local government, employment, the police and health (Pratchett, 2004). It is also embedded in the political discourse of both government and opposition parties as demonstrated by suggestions in 2006 for an independent NHS Board, a BBC style constitution for the NHS that sets out a central framework with freedom for NHS organisations to develop local approaches and Conservative Party proposals for an independent NHS (BBC News, 23 September, 2006; Burnham, 2006; *Guardian*, 9 October, 2006).

Yet while decentralisation appears to be back in fashion there is still a strong centralist theme to government health policy such as the reaction in England to NHS deficits and ensuring financial balance leading to increased central intervention in NHS Trusts (including job cuts) and Primary Care Trusts (PCTs) (where mergers have been imposed). There is also an acknowledgement that more central control may be required with evolving regulatory processes and new central regulatory bodies (including mergers of existing ones), in England, Wales and Scotland, to ensure NHS performance improves.

Given the continuing strength of centralist interventions it is important to question, therefore, to what extent the NHS is decentralising and what form this takes. However, decentralisation is an ill defined concept and while there are existing conceptual frameworks these present a number of problems when applied in practice – raising questions about their relevance in general and their usefulness when applied to the NHS. This chapter examines these questions and draws on a review of the evidence on the organisational performance impact of decentralisation in the English NHS undertaken for the National Co-ordinating Centre for Service Development and Organisation (Peckham et al., 2005). Focusing on the experience in England we apply a new analytical framework for examining decentralisation and centralisation. The first section of this chapter examines existing frameworks and introduces the Arrows Framework. This is followed by a discussion of current health care policy applying the framework to highlight the potential problems and pitfalls in formulating and implementing this decentralist approach.

Conceptualising Decentralisation

Decentralisation is a complex concept and is used in a wide range of disciplinary contexts but while primarily defined as a spatial, organisational or political concept it remains a contested concept lacking clarity of definition (Smith, 1985; Peckham et al., 2007). Decentralisation is associated with the development of the 'new public management' as part of the shift from the constraints of working with an old-fashioned 'public administrative' bureaucracy (Hoggett, 1996; Powell, 1998; Ferlie et al., 1997, New Public Management). A number of studies have examined the process of decentralisation, or theorise it and present its advantages and disadvantages but offer little evidence to support the claims for improvement in services made for decentralisation (Bossert, 1996; Burns et al., 1994; Peckham et al., 2005). Discussion and analysis of decentralisation has relied on a limited number heuristic frameworks which are briefly mentioned here but are more fully discussed elsewhere by Peckham et al. (2005, 2007).

The most widely used framework is Rondinelli's which defines four dimensions of decentralisation (1981): de-concentration reflecting a shift in authority, delegation where semi-autonomous agencies are granted new powers, devolution represented by a shift in authority to state, provincial or municipal governments and privatisation. Studies of decentralisation on UK local government and the civil service (Burns et al., 1994; Hambleton et al., 1996; Pollitt et al., 1998) also identify similar also established dimensions such as localisation, flexibility, devolved, organisational and democratisation (Burns et al., 1994); geography-based, power-based, managerial, political (Hambleton et al., 1996); politics, competitive and internal (Pollitt et al., 1998). These frameworks reflect concepts of horizontal, spatial dispersal and vertical movement between political and administrative layers (Smith, 1985). Decentralisation as defined in these frameworks can therefore only be seen in relation to a specific set of circumstances or by comparison to some other state i.e. centralisation.

Bossert (1998) has suggested a further approach based on a principal/agent framework as this takes into consideration the relationship between central and local authorities – those giving power or authority and those in receipt of it – which sets the decentralist/centralist relationship. He links this to an analysis of 'decision space – the 'range of effective choice' organisations or individuals have. For Bossert a key characteristic of decentralisation is that any discretion or autonomy is dependent on being given by a higher authority. Bossert also draws attention to local fiscal choice which is based on the assumption that decentralisation gives agencies resource raising powers creating fiscal federalism (Oates, 1972; Smith, 1985). This does not apply to the UK NHS as budgets are centrally set with little if any local revenue raising. Another approach is social capital drawing on Putnam's work and linking decentralisation to concepts of community involvement and participation (Bossert, 1998; Putnam, 2000). However, the premise here is that decentralisation will only be effective in areas with established social and civic networks. Bossert (1998) argues such an approach is not useful although he acknowledges that studies of decentralization should take the local context into account. However, a key problem with these frameworks is that they tend to be over simplistic and applying them as an analytical framework meets a number of problems (Peckham et al., 2007). These are:

1. Problems of clarity: leading to a substantial variation in how the concept is applied (Peckham et al., 2005). As Mintzberg (1979) has argued – decentralization 'remains probably the most confused topic in organization theory' while de Vries (2000) notes that many of the claims made for the benefits of decentralisation can also be made for centralisation (see also Walker, 2003).
2. Problems of terminology: failing to clarify what particular aspect of the process of government is 'decentralised' due to using imprecise terms. Concepts such as power and authority or delegation and devolution are also conflated. Confusion of what might constitute a mode of organisation rather than decentralisation per se is evidenced by Rondinelli's inclusion of privatisation – essentially the lateral dispersion at particular organisational levels – more akin to the concept of hollowing out (Rhodes, 1997) or fragmentation (Boyne, 1992).
3. Problems of context: meaning that the frameworks are highly contextual in terms of time and place and do not capture the complexity of government; transferability and generalisability are thus limited. Application to the NHS is often difficult as frameworks are relevant to local government and democratic political contexts, or involve revenue raising powers. Frameworks do not address the inter and intra-organisational aspects evident in current debates about the NHS and public services more generally.
4. Problems of scope: emphasis is placed on decentralisation from national government to provincial/regional/local government, overlooking the potential for decentralisation to individuals and/or centralisation beyond the nation state. In other words, only a limited part of the centralization-decentralization spectrum tends to be used. Debates about the 'hollowing out' of, or 'congested state' (Rhodes, 1997; Skelcher, 2000; Pollitt and Talbot, 2004) indicate a broader process at work rather than simply examining a local/central relationship. Existing frameworks fail to capture the shift of power upward and downwards and are also locked in an organisational frame ignoring the individual patient, manager, clinician or citizen.
5. Problems of operationalisation and measurement: offering little indication of how to operationalise decentralisation as an analytical concept. Most frameworks are typologies or lists, and do not give much assistance in comparison of decentralisation beyond nominal categories.

The Arrows Framework

In order to overcome these problems we have developed a new framework that draws on a wider conceptualisation of the levels of decentralisation – "from where to where", allows an explicit recognition of both centralising and decentralising processes and which draws on the organisational and management literature categorisation of organisations and their activities. In the framework the "from where to where" question is conceptualised in terms of the aggregation or disaggregation of population so that:

Decentralisation = towards more disaggregation (more individual autonomy)

Centralisation = towards more aggregation (groupings of individuals or organisations and less individual autonomy).

The next question is to examine how is it possible to provide a contextual framework that can address the what of decentralisation? Our suggestion is that given that the performance literature uses a configuration of inputs, process and outcomes (IPO) that it is useful to apply these as the second (vertical axis) dimension of the framework (Hales, 1999; Boyne, 2002). This configuration is also widely used in the management, economics and organisational literature as a method of categorisation (Sheaff et al., 2004). This is simply a categorical device – one could use other configurations such as logistics, commissioning or human resources, or responsibility/accountability and authority. However, the use of IPO configuration provides a way of disaggregating activities, functions or policies to examine their impact on any particular level or element of the framework's horizontal axis. Thus a simple two dimensional framework would like the following which we are calling the Arrows Framework shown in Figure 3.1 applied in a UK health care context:

Levels → Activity ↓	Global	Europe	UK	England/ Scotland/ Wales/ Northern Ireland	Region Eg. Strategic Health Authorities	Organisation Eg. Primary Care Trust	Sub-unit Eg. Locality/ GP practice	Individual professional/ practitioner	Individual patient
Inputs	Direction of movement ←——→								
Process	Direction of movement ←——→								
Outcomes	Direction of movement ←——→——→								

Figure 3.1 Decentralisation – Arrows Framework

The framework provides a way of plotting movements and directions between organisational and spatial levels – from individuals to populations and vice versa along the different dimensions of what is being centralised/decentralised. The framework, in itself, does not say whether such movements lead to particular configurations of power or to specific transfer of responsibility, authority or power, however, it does provide a way of identifying the pattern of movement – centralising and decentralising and sets a framework for examining inter-relationships between such movements.

Using the IPO configuration it is possible to plot movements of decentralisation/centralisation. While the allocation of inputs, processes and outcomes is clearly open to some interpretation it should be possible to develop agreement about such categories or at least in application provide justification for allocating policies or functions to one of the categories. However, applying this approach to the NHS it is possible to allocate finance, resources, skills, organisational form and structure etc as inputs; commissioning, service delivery, governance as processes and performance targets (specifying things to be achieved), inspection (as a final assessment of performance of organisations such as that by the Healthcare Commission) etc. as outcomes. However, as this structure mainly provides a way of plotting both the direction of transfer and different functions that can be actions or policies concern about actual categorisation may be less important than disaggregating the different functions or policies in a way that demonstrates different movements across the framework. Some functions or activities are easy to categorise funding and staffing are clear service inputs, commissioning is clearly a process and performance targets and measurement are outcomes. Others are more complex – is patient choice process (the process of choice) or outcome (having a choice)? Also what outcomes? For patients or for the health system? Figure 3.2 demonstrates how inputs into patient choice have become more decentralised but there are more actors in the process reflecting funding, service organisation, provision and acquisition of advice and information. Categorisation may, therefore, be open to challenge although it is possible that whether the more complex activities sit as input, process or outcome may be less important than identifying their direction of travel and that they are seen as one of a number of activities as shown in Figure 3.2.

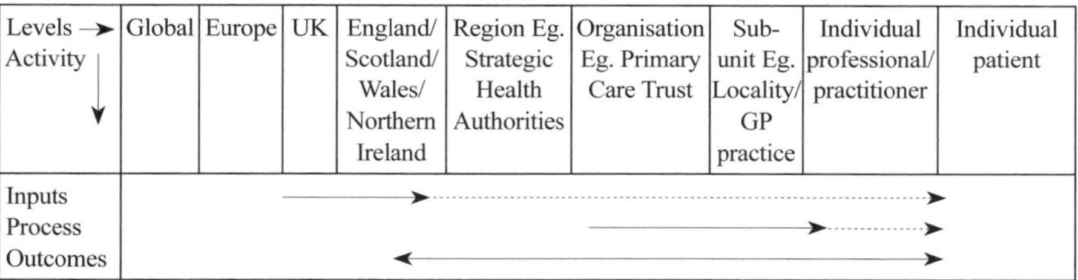

Levels → Activity ↓	Global	Europe	UK	England/ Scotland/ Wales/ Northern Ireland	Region Eg. Strategic Health Authorities	Organisation Eg. Primary Care Trust	Sub-unit Eg. Locality/ GP practice	Individual professional/ practitioner	Individual patient
Inputs									
Process									
Outcomes									

Figure 3.2 Decentralisation – Patient Choice Policy in England

To use the Arrows Framework effectively the start and end points and length of each arrow is significant for each component (inputs, process and outcomes). Each table can be read vertically, e.g. the arrows demonstrate the effect on each hierarchical level (e.g. region, PCT) as well movements (centralisation/decentralisation) within particular functions or polices. This allows comparison between levels and components and demonstrates that centralisation and decentralisation can occur simultaneously highlighting the ambiguity of the concepts and a factor missing from previous decentralisation frameworks. The collective direction of arrows would demonstrate more decentralisation/ centralisation – although it is not clear whether having the arrows all moving in one direction is more supportive or disruptive. The framework can be vertically transected at any particular point to examine the relative directions of the arrows and whether this is the start, middle or end point of each arrow – providing a picture of the intersection between any particular point on the lateral dimension and specific policies or activities being decentralised or centralised. While the framework identifies the direction and extent of decentralisation/ centralisation it cannot show what this means in terms of the discretion or latitude this brings at any point – the room for manoeuvre of any individual or organisation (Bossert, 1998; Exworthy and Frosini, 2006). However, the ability to demonstrate the extent and direction is useful in terms of being able to provide the basis for a more detailed analysis of decentralisation.

Decentralisation and the NHS: Current Contexts

The NHS embodies both diversity and uniformity. Within a national health service that is (notionally) committed to equity, the pressures for uniformity appear strong. The national (UK) character of the health service is reinforced by central funding and an emphasis on shared values such as equitable access, universality, free access etc as well as professional conformity and common standards or conditions of service (Hunter and Wistow, 1987). However, it is possible to identify a series of local health services (Powell, 1998) and this diversity might provide locally contingent services and local horizontal integration (Exworthy and Peckham, 1998) but it may also lead to inequality and fragmentation (Peckham and Exworthy, 2003). Butler (1992: 125) summarises the dichotomy: is the NHS a national service which is locally managed or a series of local services operating within national guidelines?

Recent pressures encouraging diversity include political devolution within the UK leading to four NHS's, territorial cultures and traditions, the way in different types of policy are implemented, the territorial regimes of governance and the restructuring of the state in the light of broader pressures (Greer, 2005). Implementation theories also highlight the need to balance professional and organisational discretion for health professionals and local NHS agencies (suggesting a devolved and decentralised organisational structure) and central policy control to achieve policy delivery (Harrison and Pollitt, 1994; Hill, 1997).

UK health policy promotes a number of broad themes that include organisational freedom from central control, patient empowerment and clinical empowerment reflecting concerns that the NHS is over centralised and over politicised and that there should be a greater distance between the NHS and government, to separate providers from central control and have greater devolution from the centre (King's Fund 2002). The policy theme of decentralization is evident across the range of most UK health policy. In England this includes the introduction of Patient Choice, Foundation Trusts, Payment by Results and Practice-Based Commissioning, among many others (DoH, 2000, 204, 2005a, 2006). In Wales the role of Local Health Boards and local networks is emphasised and in Scotland new powers are being developed for local Community Health Partnerships (WAG, 2005; SEHD, 2005).

In England the goals of this current round of decentralisation appear to be threefold:

1. to stimulate a self-sustaining set of incentives which foster continuous organisational reform;

2. to allow greater autonomy but on a selective basis and dependent on central assessment of performance against centrally set criteria;
3. to create a pluralist model of local provision (DoH, 2006).

The purchaser-provider distinction (first created in the 1990s quasi-market) is being extended to allow new market entrants from the for-profit and not for profit sectors. This is not a passive process but one that has been actively encouraged. For example, Patient Choice policy requires patients to be given a choice of 4–5 providers, one of whom had to be a private/independent organization. This compares with the approach in Wales where patient choice is a centrally driven programme aimed at reducing waiting lists.

Local services have been at the heart of the NHS since its inception – note the concepts of local GPs and local hospitals. This emphasis on decentralised service provision has remained a strong feature of the UK NHS. Increasingly questions about the quality and uniformity of services across the country have surfaced alongside concerns about post code lottery in accessing services. The centre/local tension is explicit in discussions of equity and quality and across the UK there is a shift towards decentralisation of control over inputs and processes but increasing centralisation of outcome measures through performance targets and regulation (Peckham et al., 2005; Peckham, 2006).

The local nature of the NHS has found form most recently in the development of primary care organisations. The development of local primary care organisations was at the heart of NHS reforms in the late 1990s – particularly in England and Wales with the creation of Primary Care Groups and then Trusts and Local Health Boards. However, in response to system pressures on finances and to strengthen commissioning there have been moves to network or merge these small PCOs during 2006. Ironically in Scotland the shift has been in the opposite direction with the formalisation and development of local Community Health Partnerships to focus local partnership work between health (especially general practice) and local authorities with the Unified Boards retaining their commissioning role (NHS Scotland, 2005). In this sense the concept of larger, rather than smaller commissioners, is a common factor across the UK demonstrating a central concern with inputs and processes through structural reorganisation. However, in England the push to a more pluralist pattern of health care provision is distinct from the approaches in Wales and Scotland and demonstrates a more dispersed system. However, whether it is right to describe this as decentralist is open to question given that funding (inputs) and performance frameworks (outcomes) remain largely centralised. Thus, by applying the Arrows Framework we would see that process aspects of health care delivery are currently in flux with the process of commissioning and provision being (centrally) reorganised creating shifts along this axis of the framework - centralising in England and Wales and decentralising in Scotland. One uniform shift is the increasing centralisation of performance frameworks with Scotland and Wales shifting to more central control of local health care organisations in terms of their outcomes (SEHD, 2005; WAG, 2005).

Patient choice is perhaps one area that would appear to clearly be decentralist in nature in England. The rhetoric of choice in welfare services has been a feature of the government's policy since its election in 1997 and since 2001 English NHS policy has been committed to allowing patients a greater say in their own health care, for example by choosing or sharing in the decision about where they should be treated, what kind of treatment to have or who should carry it out decentralising decisions further than simply to local NHS organizations and professionals. This represents a shift towards greater consumerism (Greener, 2004). Greater patient choice, outlined in various policy documents (DoH, 2000, 2003, 2004, 2005a), has been supported by professional and consumer groups although it is widely acknowledged that there are limits to, and adverse consequences of, choice (NCC, 2004; Fotaki et al., 2005). However, choice is not a uniform policy across the UK and while this consumerist model is most developed within England, in Wales the current emphasis on choice (Second Offer System) is driven very centrally and focused specifically as a management tool to meet national waiting time targets (Welsh Assembly Government, 2005). Neither is it entirely clear that all aspects of patient choice represent decentralisation as shown in Figure 3.2. Payment by results and developing a more pluralistic system of health care providers go hand in hand with patient choice with competition and contestability as key drivers for improving health care services to meet centrally defines outcomes. Similarly, public health policy and the increasing emphasis on self care sets out a strategy based on individual responsibility and rights and obligations to others with state intervention (e.g. banning smoking in public places or providing support services such as information and equipment) only where necessary (DoH, 2005b, 2006).

However, there have been countervailing centrist policy shifts with the imposition of national contracts for consultants, centrally negotiated provider contracts, rationalisation of PCTs and Strategic Health Authorities in England and the centralisation and concentration of performance monitoring in the Healthcare Commission. The emphasis on targets (especially in England) has ensured that performance of the NHS is centrally driven – a situation that is increasingly pertinent in the other home countries. In addition the continuing development of National Service Frameworks, evidence based medicine and national guidelines (from NICE in England and Wales and NHS Quality Improvement Scotland) – and the way decisions in one part of the UK spill over across all parts of the UK (see recent debates about herceptin), emphasise the importance of central approaches to standard setting that can restrict individual professional freedoms to practice and local variations in service delivery. Interestingly some aspects of health care demonstrate both centralist and decentralist approaches. For example, national pay agreements such as Agenda for Change and the application of the Knowledge Skills Framework and approaches to workforce allocation, education and training are on the one hand centralised through national negotiation and agreement, workforce planning etc but involve local decisions about using frameworks to develop local innovative solutions, change work force patterns etc.

What is clear is that the traditional decentralisation frameworks do not provide a useful way of examining the complex shifts of decentralisation and centralisation in contemporary UK health policy. These frameworks require a single concept of decentralisation – and do not provide a way of capturing multiple movements in different directions. In contrast the application of the Arrows Framework does provide initial approach that helps to examine this complexity. Each of these organisational/

policy changes described above has a distinct centralist or decentralist flavour that can be analysed within the Arrows Framework reflecting shifts along the inputs, processes and outcomes dimensions. In addition at a policy level it is possible to map the countervailing directions of health policy and to identify multiple directions of travel in terms of centralising and decentralising policies – and in some cases decentralising and centralising policy such as payment by results where tariffs are set nationally but patient flows are determined locally (rather than PCT negotiated contracts). In comparison the frameworks discussed earlier in this paper would not have captured the nuances of this and therefore the extension of the framework's lateral axis and the categorisation of activities or policies into IPO facilitates a more sensitive analysis.

Above all the framework helps us understand the complexity and ambiguity of current health policy. By examining policies and changes through an IPO configurations and an extended centralisation-decentralisation spectrum the framework can start to unpack both intended and unintended consequences and the effects on individual agencies or people or levels of government. Policy creates uncertainty and complexity by extending the range of actors through decentralisation patient choice is a good example of this as choice is framed by decisions made at national, local, professional and individual patient levels. The implications of decentralisation in one area can also be compared with impacts on another. For example if decentralisation is an approach to deliver greater organisational efficiency, what are the effects on inequality? There is bound to be a trade off between these (Peckham et al., 2005). Here again we can use patient choice policy to explore whether there will be greater or less equity at any point on the framework (Fotaki et al., 2005).

In determining whether patient choice is truly decentralist it is necessary to examine how the policy works and the Arrows Framework does provide a useful way of conceptualising this. Rhetorically there is decentralisation to individual choice but patients often defer to the GP as proxy and the extent of consumerism may be minimised by professional deference (Fotaki et al., 2005). The London patient choice pilots highlighted the important role of practices in assisting and supporting patient choice and it is not clear how far this actually influences choices made (ibid.). In addition, the information informing patient choice decisions (by patients or GPs) may be shaped by informal and formal performance (outcome) measures (such as HCC annual health check or local media reports). Hence the IPO configurations do not exist in isolation but rather are dynamic and synergistic and the decentralisation of choice is not, therefore necessarily to the patient but is an area contextualised by patient/practice interactions. However, there is a real shift as by giving patients and GPs more room for manoeuvre, it may have the effect of minimising the decision space of other organisations (e.g. Trusts) depending on their and the PCT's ability in demand management – setting the context within which choices are made (Ferlie et al., 2006).

Conclusion

Developments in health policy and health services organisation and delivery in the UK create a complex pattern of shifts both between different actors or levels within the health system, but also within each level. Current policy and organisational changes highlight the need to engage with concepts of decentralisation that move beyond the simple organisational context and which capture changes in government relations and also incorporate an individual context. They also demonstrate the simultaneous nature of centralist and decentralist movements in policy and activities and the only conclusion that is possible about whether the NHS is decentralising is to yes it is and no it is not. Clearly devolution to Northern Ireland, Scotland and Wales has created a new context and a more devolved NHS (not one but four NHSs) but within these four NHS there are both strong centralising tendencies for uniformity, regulation, performance etc as well as decentralist approaches to health care delivery. Government policy rhetoric promotes decentralisation as a way of releasing local health services from the constraint of central direction and has underpinned the drive towards improvements in health care (King's Fund, 2002; DoH, 2000; DoH, 2004). Such arguments have been central to debates about independent boards and constitutions but there is little evidence to support decentralisation as contributing to organisational and health system performance (Sheaff et al., 2004; Peckham et al., 2005). Thus the inherent tension of local versus central is likely to remain a key contested arena for many years to come. In future what may become of increasing interest is the extent to which the devolved systems of the NHS themselves create a centralist, rather than decentralist, impetus to policy development in each of the four countries due to institutionalist and political pressures for uniformity. The Arrows Framework, and this analysis of UK health policy may also provide lessons for other countries and non health policy – although the nature of IPO configurations, form of decentralisation and nature of individual need will have to be contextualised for the different circumstances.

Acknowledgements

This chapter is based on research undertaken for the National Co-ordinating Centre for Service Delivery and Organisation R&D, SDO-67-2003. Decentralisation as an organisational model for health care in England.

References

Bossert,T. (1996), 'Decentralization', (Chapter 9, pp. 147–159) in *Health Policy and systems development: an agenda for research*. Edited by K. Janovsky, World Health Organization, Geneva.

Bossert, T.J. (1998), 'Analyzing the decentralization of health systems in developing countries: decision space, innovation, and performance', *Social Science and Medicine*, **47**(10), 1513–1527.

Boyne, G. (1992), 'Local government structure and performance: lessons from America?' *Public Administration*, **70**, 333–357.

Boyne, G. (2002), 'Concepts and Indicators of Local Authority Performance: An Evaluation of the Statutory Frameworks in England and Wales', *Public Money and Management*, **22**(2), 17–24.

Burnham, A. (September 2006), 'A Health Constitutional Progress', http://progressonline.org.uk/Magazine/article.aspa=1399.

Burns, D., Hambleton, R. and Hoggett, P. (1994), *The Politics of Decentralisation*, Macmillan, Basingstoke.

Butler, J. (1992), *Patients, Policies and Politics*, Open University Press, Buckingham.

Department of Health (1997), *The New NHS*, TSO, London.

Department of Health (2000), *The NHS Plan*. London.

Department of Health (2003), *Building on the Best: Choice, Responsiveness and Equity in the NHS*, London.

Department of Health (2004), *The NHS Improvement Plan: Putting People at the Heart of Public Services*. London.

Department of Health (2005a), *Creating a Patient led NHS: Delivering the NHS Improvement Plan*, London.

Department of Health (2005b), *Delivering Choosing Health: Making Healthier Choices Easier*, London.

Department of Health (2006), *Our Health, Our Care, Our Say*, Cm. 6737 TSO, London.

De Vries, M. (2000), 'The rise and fall of decentralization: A comparative analysis of arguments and practices in European countries', *European Journal of Political Research*, **38**, 193–224.

Exworthy, M. and Frosini, F. (2006), 'Room to manoeuvre? Explaining the impact of English health policies upon local autonomy', Paper presented to the PSA/SPA 'Health politics' conference, Oxford, August 2006.

Exworthy, M. and Peckham, S. (1998), 'The contribution of coterminosity to joint purchasing health and social care', *Health and Place*, **4**(3), 233–243.

Ferlie, E., Freeman, G., McDonnell, J., Petsoulas, C. and Rundle-Smith, S. (2006), 'Introducing Choice in the Public Services: Some Supply-Side Issues', *Public Money and Management*, **26**(1), 63–72.

Fotaki, M., Boyd, A., Smith, L., McDonald, R., Roland, M., Sheaff, R., Edwards, A. and Elwyn, G. (2005), *Patient Choice and the Organisation and Delivery of Health Services: Scoping Review Manchester*, University of Manchester.

Greener, I. (2004), 'The three moments of New Labour's health policy discourse', *Policy and Politics*, **32**(3) 303–316.

Hales, C. (1999), 'Leading horses to water? The impact of decentralization on managerial behaviour', *Journal of Management Studies*, **36**(6), 831–851.

Hambleton, R. and Hoggett, P. (1987), *Decentralisation and Democracy: Localising Public Services*, SAUS, Bristol.

Harrison, S. and Pollitt, C. (1994), *Controlling Health Professionals*, Open University Press, Buckingham.

Healthcare Commission (2005), *State of Healthcare 2005 London*.

Hill, M. (1997), 'Implementation theory: yesterday's issue', *Policy and Politics*, **25**(4), 275–385.

Hoggett, P. (1996), 'New modes of control in the public sector', *Public Administration*, **74**, 9–32.

Hudson, B. (1999), 'Decentralisation and Primary Care Groups: a paradigm shift for the NHS in England?', *Policy and Politics*, **27**(2), 159–172.

Hunter, D.J. and Wistow, G. (1987), *Community Care in Britain: Variations on a Theme*, King Edward's Hospital Fund for London, London.

Hutton W. (2000), New Life for Health: *The Commission on the NHS*, Virago, London.

King's Fund (2002), 'The future of the NHS: A framework for debate', Discussion paper, January 2002, Haskins Report, London.

Klein, R. (2001), *The New Politics of the NHS*, (4th edn), Pearson, Harlow.

Klein, R. (2003), 'The new localism? Once more through the revolving door?', *Journal of Health Services Research and Policy*, **8**(4), 195–196.

Levaggi, R. and Smith, P.C. (2004), 'Decentralization in health care: Lessons from public economics', Unpublished paper, York University.

Mintzberg, H. (1979), *The Structuring of Organizations*, Prentice Hall, New York.

National Consumer Council 2004, 'Making public services personal: a new compact for public services NCC', London.

NHS Scotland (2005), 'The national framework for service change in NHS Scotland: elective care action team – final report', SEHD, Edinburgh.

Oates, W.E. (1972), *Fiscal federalism*, Harcourt Brace Jovanovich, New York.

Osborne, D. and Gaebler, T. (1992), *Reinventing Government: How the Entrepreneurial Spirit Is Transforming The Public Sector*, Addison-Wesley, Reading.

Peckham S. (2007), 'One or Four? The NHS in 2006', in Clarke K., *Social Policy Review*, **19**, Policy Press, Bristol.

Peckham, S. and Exworthy, M. (2003), *Primary Care in The UK: Policy, Organisation and Management*, Palgrave MacMillan, Basingstoke.

Peckham, S., Exworthy, M., Powell, M. and Greener, I. (2005), *Decentralisation as an Organisational Model for Health Care in England*, NCCSDO, London.

Peckham, S., Exworthy, M., Powell, M. and Greener, I. (2007), 'Decentralisation in health care: A new conceptual framework', *Public Administration*.

Pollitt, C., Brichall, J. and Putnam, K. (1998), *Decentralising Public Service Management*, Macmillan, London.

Pollitt C. and Talbot, C. (eds) (2004), *Unbundled Government – A Critical Analysis of the Global Trend to Agencies, Quangos and Contracting*, Routledge, London.

Powell, M. (1998), 'In what sense a National Health Service', *Public Policy and Administration*, **13**(3), 56–69.

Pratchett, L. (2004), 'Local autonomy, local democracy and the "New Localism"', *Political Studies*, **52**, 358–375.

Putnam, R. (2000), *Bowling Alone: The Collapse and Revival of American Community*, Simon and Schuster, New York.

Rhodes, R.A.W. (1997), *Understanding Governance: Policy Networks, Governance, Reflexivity and Accountability*, Open University Press, Buckingham.

Rondinelli, D.A. (1983), 'Implementing decentralization programmes in Asia: A comparative analysis', *Public Administration and Development*, **3**(3), 181–207.

Sheaff, R., Schofield, J., Mannion, R., Dowling, B., Marshall, M.N. and McNally, R. (2004), *Organisational Factors and Performance: A Review of the Literature*, NCCSDO, London.

Skelcher, C. (2000), 'Changing images of the state: overloaded, hollowed-out', congested, *Public Policy and Administration*, **15**(3), 3–19.

Smith, B.C. (1985), *Decentralization: The Territorial Dimension of the State*, Allen and Unwin, London.

Vancil, R.F. (1979), *Decentralization: Managerial Ambiguity by Design*, Dow Jones Irwin, Illinois.

Welsh Assembly Government (2005), 'Designed for Life: Creating World Class Health and Social Care for Wales in the 21st Century', *Wales Assembly Government*, Cardiff.

Chapter 4

Modernising Health Policy Making

Arturo Alvarez-Rosete

Modernising the UK Government[1]

The UK policy process has changed profoundly over the last two decades. The former Westminster/Whitehall model of the policy process in which policies were almost exclusively drafted by civil servants who then submitted them to ministers for their approval before being introduced in Parliament – all taking place in a closed environment, isolated from major external influences – has been criticised as an inappropriate description for current British politics and policy processes. 'Governance', instead of the old style of 'government', has instead been suggested as a concept which 'sensitises us to the numerous actors, the variety of terrains and the different relationships involved in the policy process of governing' (Richards and Smith, 2002: 19; Pierre and Peters, 2000; Rhodes 1997).

The policy process is now crowded with more and new actors such as delivery agencies, international organisations (the European Union) and new social groups such as health consumer groups (Baggott et al., 2004), while the government is not necessarily the most powerful actor in the policy arena. Ministers and civil servants engage with other actors, exchanging resources and thus establishing stable patterns of interaction in the form of 'policy networks'. Globalisation, 'europeanization', devolution and decentralisation (to local authorities and arm's length bodies) have opened up policy making arenas which were previously limited to the central government level.

Policy making therefore takes place now in a substantially different setting – one which is more fragmented and even messier than before. Arguably, this 'balkanisation of public policy making' (Wright and Hayward, 2000), in part a result of previous managerial reforms (Newman, 2001), is undermining the ability of central government to make policy and control the policy arena (Richards and Smith, 2002).

The British Labour Government elected in 1997, reacted to these governance challenges by launching, in 1999, a programme for modernising the machinery and practices of government that could rebuild some central government capacity, developing new coordination mechanisms and making government more responsive to the public. The 1999 Cabinet Office *Modernising Government* White Paper and

1 I would like to thank Jo Maybin, Nicholas Mays and Anthony Harrison for their helpful comments on earlier drafts of this chapter and all participants at the Politics of Health Group Annual Conference in Oxford in September 2005.

the subsequent documents and initiatives that followed (see Table in Appendix for a selection of key documents), in particular the 1999 Cabinet Office report *Professional Policy Making for the 21st Century*, suggested a model of 'modern' policy-making based on three 'themes': vision, effectiveness and continuous improvement. The themes were then translated into nine 'core competencies': forward looking; outward looking; innovative and creative; evidence-based; inclusive; joined up; uses evaluation; employs reviews; and learns lessons.

The degree to which the 'Modernising Government' agenda is underpinned by a coherent governance theory is the subject for discussion. For Newman, despite her conclusion that overall, the Labour reforms actually reflect an overlapping of different styles, the model at least seems to be embedded in the language of the Governance literature and to advocate 'a new network-based style of governance' (Newman, 2001: 64). However, Parsons (2001) argues that the Cabinet Office model only reflects an 'awareness' of the governance narrative and fails to integrate the conditions of fragmentation and complexity in which current policy making takes place.

Modernising Policy Making at the Department of Health

The Cabinet Office report *Professional Policy Making for the 21st Century* report audited cases identified by departments themselves as examples of good policy making practice. The overall conclusion was that government departments were improving their policy making practice in areas such as joining up work, involving those affected by policies and implementers and outward learning (from other countries). However, the audit also revealed a lack of good practice in developing a forward-looking vision, being innovative and creative, basing policies on sound evidence and learning lessons from past experience.

Although the report included a few examples from the Department of Health (DH), there has been no systematic assessment of the quality of policy making at the DH in England or of whether it has succeeded in 'modernising' its policy making style. This chapter aims to contribute to filling that gap.

There are signs of improvement and examples of good practice policy making at the DH, as well as evidence of a true commitment on the part of policy makers to improve the quality of their work. Departmental organisational changes have brought about a more streamlined department with new structures and new policy making styles (Alvarez-Rosete, 2004). A departmental Regulatory Impact Unit has been set up. A Policy Hub has been set up to envisage new ways of improving policy formulation. For example, the Policy Hub has explored a new methodology for developing policy through the Policy Collaborative experiment. The aim of the Policy Collaborative is to develop policy through the continuous involvement of frontline staff and stakeholders. The core of the policy making work is done by teams formed by DH civil servants, supported by a project facilitator, who are in charge of developing policy in selected areas - from long-term illnesses to transplants, cancer or developing NHS standards. Each team is required to work with at least 30 external stakeholders (Alvarez-Rosete, 2005).

Since April 2003, the DH has been applying the Office of Government Commerce-sponsored Gateway Project Review Process to all high-risk and medium-risk investment projects undertaken by the department, NHS and arms' length bodies. The process consists of a series of short peer reviews at key stages of a program or project in partnership with the project team and stakeholders to identify potential risks and implementation problems.

A former Chief Economist at the DH, Clive Smee asserts that the quality of health policy making in England has improved as it has become more evidence based and rigorous (Smee, 2005) and, although 'there is still much further to go', it has taken on more of the characteristics of a 'learning organisation' (Smee, 2006: 2). Also, according to Larsen et al. (2006), the DH policy making in long-term care has evolved into a much more inclusive style.

However, contemporary discussion of NHS policy making tends to point to the high degree of central political control over the initiation and development of policy. A 2002 King's Fund paper considered over-politicisation, excessive centralisation and lack of responsiveness to individuals and local communities to be the most immediate obstacles to the effective management of the NHS (King's Fund, 2002) and these criticisms (with the consequent proposal of creating an independent NHS agency at arm's length) surfaced again during the round of political party conferences in Autumn 2006.

Commentators have pointed to a lack of coherence in recent health policies and reforms (Harding, 2005), politicians' obsession with micro-managing health services (Greer, 2005) and the strains placed on the health service by the large number of centrally-driven targets and the constant flux of radical policies and reforms. Referring to the policy making styles in the four UK administrations, Jervis and Plowden (2003) suggest that in Wales, Scotland and Northern Ireland there are higher levels of openness, inclusiveness and transparency than in England.

Some of the very recent departmental reforms (in 2006) may reinforce these negative perceptions. Interestingly, the announcement of a 'rapid review' of the Department's analytical capacity and organisational arrangements may suggest an alarming absence of analytical capability at the Department.

In sum, there is circumstantial evidence of progress and examples of good practice, but the 'popular' image that persists is that of a close, reactive policy process in which policies are not based on sound evidence. Thus, there is a need for systematic research on whether there have been any improvements in the quality of health policy making at the DH in England.

Evaluating the Quality of Policy Making at the DH

This chapter reports the evaluation of the DH's policy making style against a standard of best practice developed from the 'Modernising Government' literature. It applies the standard against two examples of recent policy formulation[2] – the drafting of

2 This is not a study of the whole policy making process but of the policy formulation stage only. Although implementation and evaluation have to be taken into account from the

the Mental Health Bill (October 1998–May 2005) and the reform of the generic medicines policy (March 1999–May 2004). These two case-studies were randomly chosen with the only prerequisite of the first being a policy which required primary legislation and the second only requiring secondary legislation, as well as looking at two quite different areas of health care. There was no prior knowledge of whether these two cases were going to reflect good or bad examples of policy making.

In October 1998, due to perceived failures in existing mental health policy, concerns with public safety and changes in contemporary patterns of mental health service provision, a committee of independent experts to advise ministers on the reform of the 1983 Mental Health Act was set up. Successive Green and White Papers and two Draft Mental Health Bills in 2002 and 2004 brought into the discussion proposals for compulsory treatment through community treatment orders, a new definition of mental disorder as well as new safeguards such as the right to independent advocacy and new bodies both to determine and monitor the use of compulsory powers. Fierce opposition by mental health stakeholders and concerns with the workability of the measures ultimately led to the abandonment of the 2004 Draft Bill in March 2006 and to the announcement of a completely new bill in November 2006.

The system of supply and reimbursement of generic medicines – those drugs marketed without a brand name – for the NHS was reviewed after a sudden increase in prices in the spring of 1999. While various options to reform the generics market, including central tendering, were considered, strong opposition to radical reforms from stakeholders and even civil servants finally led the Department to leave existing procurement arrangements intact but create a statutory price control scheme and other instruments to obtain information on the performance of the market.

This research builds upon the Cabinet Office literature to propose a more comprehensive model of policy making which envisages a 'Governance' approach to the understanding of the British policy process. In the model proposed, some of the *Professional Policy Making for the 21st Century* 'core competencies' were merged and a new one which was not previously considered - the level of transparency in the process and the accountability of policy makers – was introduced. In total, the model examines eight core competencies: proactive; inclusive; joined up; forward/outward looking; evidence based; provisions for implementation; provisions for evaluation; democratic/accountable.

The eight competencies embody in themselves several dimensions. For example, 'pro-activeness' is used to denote features such as being innovative or creative as well as being anticipative and able to properly assess risks. The 'accountable/democratic' label refers to a policy making style which is transparent and open, where policy makers are accessible, there is feedback to those who participate in consultations and debates in Parliament ensure that the policy satisfies basic democratic principles. As a result of an extensive review of the literature produced by the UK government, each competency was operationalised by developing a number of measurable indicators taken from the Cabinet Office documents. In this sense, this exercise is about asking

early stages of policy making, time constraints limited the assessment to the design stages of the two policies.

whether the government is meeting their own goals and expectations. Overall, 39 indicators were produced (see Appendix).

Being based on a best practice model that the government set for itself, this evaluation of the government's health policy making becomes automatically justified in that it uses the government's own evaluation criteria and might not therefore need any further justifications. However, this might look quite cynical given the criticisms that the 'Modernising Government' model has received - and indeed any normative attempt to improve the quality of the policy making process can easily be depicted as an inherently naïve exercise which ignores the complexity and messiness of the real world. Parsons (2001) has strongly criticised the Cabinet Office model as an old-fashioned, top-down, technocratic attempt to improve policy making along the lines of the 'rational planning' theories of the 1960s and 1970s. He claims that the model ignores current approaches in public management on issues of learning, uncertainty, chaos and complexity. However, Parsons has built his arguments on the basis of reviewing a single document the 1999 Cabinet Office report *Professional Policy Making for the 21st Century*, which is problematic since it means he fails to acknowledge important improvements to the model which were introduced in subsequent documents. For example, changes were made to the core competencies of evidence-based, joined-up or evaluation.

It is not possible to deal satisfactorily in just a few paragraphs with all the dimensions and arguments in which the 'rational versus incremental' debate has been muddling itself since the early days of the public policy discipline. Instead, I would rather list the key assumptions used in this research. First, I agree with Peter John (John, 1998) that this is a 'false debate' as decision-making can be rational at certain stages and incremental at others. In this understanding, the standard used here hopes to assess and reinforce the elements that bring rationality, order and good practice into what is otherwise a very complex and messy process. Secondly, it does not predicate a linear process nor prescribes a fixed sequence for the core competencies and related strategies. Implementation and evaluation have to be considered even at the stage at which policy is formulated. Evidence is understood as dynamic and should inform the whole process of policy development. The same holds true for the dimensions of accountability or joined-up working.

Thirdly, contained in this model is a particular understanding of what a 'successful policy process' implies. Best practice could be defined in terms of the outcomes of policy – a good process produces 'good' health policies that lead to better health outcomes. Or it could be defined in technocratic (the process is rational, goal-oriented) or legalistic terms (the process has followed all the previously established procedures and stages). However, these approaches do not necessarily capture the core of the problem; we are attempting to assess the quality of a *public* process, a process through which democratically elected authorities make decisions (that imply values) over the allocation of scarce public resources. The model for best practice policy making used here cannot be understood outside a democratic political system and cannot be understood without politics and power. Policies are therefore subject to discussion, bargaining and accommodation between actors. Politics matters. However, as there cannot be a democratic and open process without some fixed rules of the game to which all players abide (a democratic process cannot be arbitrary), a good process is also one which has correctly followed the established mechanisms and rules (the legal approach). It is precisely those mechanisms and rules what guarantee the process to be fully democratic. The accountability/transparency competency has been added precisely to reflect this understanding.

Last but not least, this model is fully embodied in a 'governance narrative' and reckons that policies are now developed through policy networks of politicians, civil servants and stakeholders in a much more fluid and complex scenario than that implied by the Whitehall/Westminster model.

The research used documentary analysis techniques and non-scheduled standardised interviews. A total of 26 interviews were conducted between February and November 2004 with key policy makers at the national government level in generic medicines and mental health (including civil servants, stakeholders and policy advisers) plus academics and other experts in health policy and British politics. Interviews aimed to collect data on the policy making process on each case study; on actors' perceptions, expectations and patterns of interaction; and on their views on how the policy making style complied with the proposed model of best practice policy making.

Pro-active

Evidence from the two case studies reveal a reactive policy making style, although concerns about potential media criticisms in mental health happened to be quite a powerful motivation for pro-activeness. A great deal of blame-avoidance attitudes in the making of generics medicines policy was found. Action to tackle the situation of the generics market was undertaken quite late, when prices of medicines had been rising for more than a year. Mechanisms of institutional inertia and self-perpetuation were at work and responsible for the failure to spot potential and *de facto* problems quickly. Regarding risk management, there is little evidence of the Department having conducted proper risk assessments on either our case studies.

Inclusive

Traditionally, organisations representing patients or carers have played a very minor role in influencing the policy process. However, in recent years, there are signs of an increasing willingness on the government's part to include patients and the public in decision-making (Baggot et al., 2004). There is a widespread feeling that policy making in health care is nowadays more inclusive than it used to be.

In the two case studies, it cannot be said that policies have developed without any public or stakeholders involvement. In mental health, a series of 'policy road-testing meetings' were held to discuss the impact of specific provisions contained in the expected legislation and the Draft Mental Health Bill, published in September 2004, was put under pre-legislative scrutiny by a Committee of both Houses, thus allowing stakeholders to raise their concerns.

The evidence suggests consultations started at a very early stage. However, the two case studied reveal a very uneven compliance with the *Code of Practice on Consultation* on the 12 week period requirement between the publication of the policy paper and the deadline for receiving stakeholders' responses. This is confirmed by the Regulatory Impact Unit's latest report on departmental compliance with the *Code of Practice on Consultation,* which concludes that only 27 out of 61 consultations carried out by the DH between January and December 2003 complied with the 12 week period required by both codes of practice – one of the worst scores among government departments (Cabinet Office, May 2004).

However, as Quennell (2001) put it, the question is not whether groups involved in the policy process are 'getting their say' but whether they are 'getting their way'. The evidence from our research is that there is a feeling of frustration among groups outside government with interests in mental health and generics medicines because they feel they are consulted but not really listened to.

Joined-up

The two case-studies revealed a growing concern for joined-up efforts among DH policymakers but also clear difficulties. In general, stakeholders perceived a lack of shared aims and objectives among departments and non-departmental public bodies. Generics policy was developed mainly by the Pharmacy and Industry Division at the DH, with occasional joined-up work with the NHS Purchase and Supply Agency (to do some forecasting and contingency planning) and the Prescription Pricing Authority. Although the Treasury was closely watching the evolution of the generics market and policy, this was not done jointly with the Department. In mental health, despite the Health Select Committee's requirements for increasing cross departmental work, the DH did not seem particularly concerned about the need to improve cross-cutting work.

Forward and Outward Looking

There has been a great deal of good practice on this core competency. DH policymakers do use scenario-planning and forecasting techniques and are quite open to learning from others' experiences. There was common agreement among our respondents that long-term budgeting currently enjoyed by the Department helped to develop a long-term policy vision.

The *Professional Policy Making for the 21st Century* report revealed that the DH makes extensive use of scenario planning. The 2001 *Better Policy Making* report quoted the DH project of long term planning for hospital beds as an example of good practice. This forward and outward looking good practice is confirmed in both generics and mental health policy.

There is, however, still room for improvement. One of the DH officials interviewed by us pointed out that 'we are not as systematic as we could be in using that information. We are looking at ways in which we can use our analytical colleagues, our economists, our statisticians and our research people more effectively'.

Evidence-based

Evidence well searched, appraised and analysed

Regarding the collection of evidence, *Professional Policy Making for the 21st Century* found examples of best practice across Whitehall. However, it found 'anecdotal evidence that little of the research commissioned by departments or other academic research was used by policymakers. There does seem to be a need to ensure that policy makers either have the skills themselves to find and interpret research data, or have access to others who have them.'

Generics reforms were grounded on an assessment of the generics market commissioned from an independent consultancy firm. Despite the criticisms it received, the report was, in terms of the quality of the scientific work, a good review of the market and a well thought out study of the reform alternatives. This, however, cannot be said of other research carried out by the Department and stakeholders. The concern was not to find evidence of what the best policy was, but to find corroboration for their negotiating positions.

Regulatory Impact Assessments: In both cases, the quality of RIAs gradually improved on key aspects: they were increasingly produced at early stages of the policy process; all options considered were discussed; a risk assessment was provided; costs and benefits were properly quantified; and they included a good account of the enforcement sanctions. Still, the absences are also noticeable. For example, in mental health, RIAs should have been produced but neither the the 1999 Green Paper nor the 2000 White Paper included an RIA.

All our respondents from the civil service regarded RIAs as a highly valuable tool. For one, RIAS 'are useful in terms of getting people to think in quite a logical ordered way about impacts, about what you are going to do and what the implications are'. However, it is striking that most stakeholders did not know what RIAs were and even those who had heard about them were not completely clear of what their purpose was.

Pilots: While there is evidence that the Department has been carrying out quite a few pilots, on, for example, electronic patient prescriptions, the IT programme, payment by results, to our knowledge, the introduction of the SMPS in generics, although properly modelled, was not piloted. Neither were pilots carried out for the Draft Mental Health Bill.

Provisions for Implementation

Good practice policy making requires that implementation of policies is well thought out and planned far from the outset. However, the degree of compliance with this requirement was appallingly low. None of the policies have had a proper 'implementation plan' when formulated. In mental health, neither the Green Paper nor the White Paper for the reform of the 1983 Mental Health Act embodied an articulated plan in which things such as, for example, the number of mental health tribunals or the resources needed were accounted for.

Only for the 2004 Draft Mental Health Bill has an implementation work stream been set up, but this confirms what the 2001 NAO report *Modern Policy Making* stated, that those required to implement and evaluate policies were consulted fairly late in the design process.

Provisions for Evaluation

There is evidence that some provisions for the annual evaluation of the schemes regulating generics medicines were included when formulating the regulations. For the new Draft Mental Health Bill, a Research and Monitoring stream has been set up to plan the monitoring of areas covered by the new Mental Health Act.

Accountable/Democratic

Public access to key decision makers and, in general, the Department's officials has also improved. However, our own experience when conducting this research was that access levels are still far from being satisfactory. It is still very difficult to find contact details for individuals on the Department's website (especially on generics medicines). When these are provided, there is no organisation chart of who does what and how a specific team is organised. And it becomes even more difficult to identify other key decision-makers, who, outside the DH, are also heavily involved in the policy process – for example, the Treasury Health Team, solicitors and Parliamentary Counsel, or the health special advisors team at Number 10.

Despite current debates on the alleged lack of power of the House of Commons Select Committees to hold the government accountable and to influence policy making, the Health Select Committee did play a relevant part in both case studies in two key aspects - in putting pressure on ministers to be more pro-active and in holding the government to account. It revealed some of the inconsistencies of the proposed legislation, forcing the government to produce a response to the Committee's reports. The revised Draft Mental Health Bill, once published, was put to a special pre-legislative Scrutiny Committee of both Houses, leading to a better informed debate on the bill.

Conclusion

Has the DH modernised its policy-making? Evidence from these two case studies, shows that progress has been uneven. The Department has taken the modernisation of policy making seriously and has substantially improved it in many aspects. It has become more inclusive than before; it has improved cross-cutting work; it applies different statistical techniques in order to plan ahead; it learns from others; it has more regularly sought an evidence-base for policy and the quality of Regulatory Impact Assessments has improved; policy makers are more easily contactable; etc.

But there are still signs of a prevalence of old practices and a hierarchical, closed and reactive policy making style. Consulting stakeholders and the public, although now assumed to be a necessary step in the policy process, does not necessarily mean listening to them. Our interviewees from outside government felt that the Department was now willing to show it is ready to listen, although they were sceptical about the extent to which this meant real inclusiveness.

There is no evidence that the Department is engaging in effective joined-up working. There is a lack of thinking about implementation during policy formulation. Policy makers are not straightforwardly visible and the lack of available data, reports and timely feedback to reflect accountability requires attention. The Department's style is still very reactive and there is a long way to go in using risk assessment techniques effectively.

Despite the observable improvements in the DH policy making style described above, groups outside government were sceptical about whether there had been positive changes and confirmed the 'popular' criticisms of policymaking in the NHS, reporting a lack of responsiveness, over-politicisation and micro-management by the Department. The overwhelming majority of respondents referred to politics and politicians interfering as the biggest obstacle to good practice policy making.

The research sheds light on the discussion in the governance literature on the ability of central government to control the policy agenda and policy making process. Central government, and civil servants and ministers at the DH, continue to be the main actor in making health policy. However, there are signs that their monopoly as shaping policy has somehow diminished. Civil servants think that a more consultative style on their part has not resulted in less confrontational attitudes from stakeholders. On the contrary, if anything, the new policy making style has brought more opportunities for stakeholders to attempt to shape the agenda by using zero-sum strategies. Increasing citizens' and interest groups' expectations of participating in decision-making, the growing complexity of policy problems, the difficulties civil servants have in controlling the policy agenda and process, the requirements for more accountability and transparency (in which the media plays a crucial part), all reflect a much more fragmented and complex policy making scenario.

Appendix

CORE COMP	INDICATOR	GENERIC MEDICINES	DRAFT MENTAL HEALTH BILL
PRO-ACTIVE	**Anticipatory or reactive**	Reactive. Blame avoidance attitudes	Proactive: but politically-driven to avoid media criticism
	Performance targets as warning indicators	No. Recent improvements	No
	Structures for actors to call for government's attention	No. Recent improvements	No
	Use of risk management techniques	No	No
INCLUSIVE	**Minimum 12 weeks for written consultation**	Only the 2001 consultation paper. None of the annual SMPS consultations nor the 2003 consultation paper	The Green Paper allowed four months
	Consultation starts early	Yes, with regard to OXERA's proposals. But this did not happen when setting up the SMPS.	Yes. However, responses to Green Paper too close to White Paper publication
	Clarity of consultation document: proposals, questions, etc. Plain language	Yes	Yes

Appendix continued

CORE COMP	INDICATOR	GENERIC MEDICINES	DRAFT MENTAL HEALTH BILL
JOINED UP	**Joined-up work with government departments and NDPBs**	Some contingency planning with NHS Purchase and Supply Agency Treasury's own monitoring agenda	Working closely with Home Office. Health Select Committee suggested a Mental Health Cabinet Sub-Committee: didn't happen
	Incentives for cross-cutting work	No	No
	Staff from other government organisations on secondments	No	To pursue personal careers, rather than cross-cutting work
	Cross-cutting budgets and pooling of resources	No	No
FORWARD AND OUTWARD LOOKING	**Intended outcomes present from beginning of policy formulation**	No. New policy goals (e.g., transparency, price-fixing prevention) were added to the first one (cutting down costs)	
	Government's priorities and long term aims taken into account	No clear strategy on what to do on generics. SMPS as a temporary measure	Critics say proposed legislation does not fit government's 'choice' agenda

Appendix continued

CORE COMP	INDICATOR		GENERIC MEDICINES	DRAFT MENTAL HEALTH BILL
FORWARD AND OUTWARD LOOKING	**Use of scenario planning, contingency planning, forecasting or similar techniques**		Yes. Strong analytical support from within DH and from outside	Yes. Strong analytical support from within DH and from outside
	Learning from other countries' experience		Yes	Yes. Stakeholders looked at types of CTOs overseas
	Evidence systematically researched, critically appraised and rigorously analysed according to explicit and transparent criteria		Mixed: good examples as well as instrumental use of evidence to back up negotiating positions	Commissioned research (literature review) on the existing MHA
	Regulatory Impact Assessments	**RIA attached**	Yes, although two more were required	Only partial RIAs for the 2002 and the 2004 Draft Bill. More RIAs required
		RIA at early stages	Mostly, yes. Improved over the years	No, very late. No RIAs for the Green and White papers
		Statement of objectives	Improved over the years	Yes
		All the options considered?	Good account of all options, including 'do nothing'	Good account of all options, including 'do nothing'

Appendix continued

CORE COMP	INDICATOR		GENERIC MEDICINES	DRAFT MENTAL HEALTH BILL
FORWARD AND OUTWARD LOOKING	Regulatory Impact Assessments	**Assessment of the risks and the counterfactual**	Non-existent or very poor risk assessments	Yes, very good
		Quantified costs thoroughly	Mostly satisfactory	Yes, very good
		Quantified benefits realistically	Benefits accounted for but not always satisfactorily quantified	Yes, good
	Pilots	**Pilots used**	No. OXERA designed a pilot, but never applied it	No
		Purpose of pilots explicit at the outset	N/A	N/A
		Enough time for the pilot	N/A	N/A
		Suitable piloting method (or mixture)	N/A	N/A
		Results publicised	N/A	N/A

Appendix continued

CORE COMP	INDICATOR	GENERIC MEDICINES	DRAFT MENTAL HEALTH BILL
PROVISIONS IMPLEMENTATION	**Implementation Plan produced**	No	No
	Implementers consulted throughout the process	Yes	Very late, through an Implementation Work Stream set up in the summer of 2004
	Process of involvement carefully planned	No	No
PROVISIONS FOR EVALUATION	**Evaluation included from early stages of the policy process**	Late: only in the 2003 consultation document. The SMPS contained provisions for evaluation	Late: the Research and Monitoring Stream
	Continuous evaluations throughout the process	Yes. The evolution of the market is now better monitored	There has been a specific 'policy road meeting' to develop ideas to monitor the Mental Health Act
ACCOUN TABLE/ DEMOCRATIC	**Accessibility and visibility of civil servants and policy makers - (e.g., full internal directory available)**	Not satisfactorily	Yes
	Communication Strategy	No	No
	Availability of data, reports, etc., and updated information	Some technical reports did not reach the public domain	Some technical reports did not reach the public been limited
ACCOUN TABLE/ DEMOCRATIC	**Feedback given to received responses when consulting**	Very late	Very late
	Involvement of Parliament: Select Committees, MPs' questions, etc.	Yes- Health Select Committee as catalyst	Yes- Health Select Committee as watchdog. Pre-Legislative Scrutiny Committee

Selected government's documents on policy making

Policy Making

Cabinet Office (1999), *Modernising Government White Paper*

Cabinet Office (1999), *Professional Policy Making for the Twenty First Century*

Cabinet Office (2001), *Better Policy-Making*

Strategy Unit (2002), *Identifying Good Practice in the Use of Programme and Project Management in Policy-Making*

NAO (2000), *Modernising Government. How the NAO are responding. A Progress Report*

NAO (2001), *Modern Policy-Making: Ensuring Policies Deliver Value for Money*

Evidence

NAO (2003), *Getting the Evidence: Using Research in Policy Making* (2003)

Risk Management

Strategy Unit (2002), *Risk: Improving Government's Capability to Handle Risk and Uncertainty*

Joined-up

Performance and Innovation Unit (2000), *Wiring it Up. Whitehall's Management of Cross-Cutting Policies and Services*

Forward-Looking

Performance and Innovation Unit (2000), *Adding it Up. Improving Analysis and Modelling in Central Government*

Participation and Consultation

Cabinet Office (2001), *Involving the Front-Line in Policy Making*

References

Alvarez-Rosete, A. (September 2004), 'Nigel gets nimble at health', *Public*, pp. 15, 18.

Alvarez-Rosete, A. (2005), 'Putting staff at the heart of strategy making', *Public*, June, pp. 13–14

Baggot, R., Allsop, J. and Jones, K. (2004), 'Representing the repressed? Health Consumer Groups and the national policy process', *Policy and Politics*, **32**(3), 317–31.

Greer, S. (2005), 'Why do Good Politics Make Bad Health Policy?', in Dawson, S. and Sausman, C. (eds), *Future Health Organisations and Systems*, Basingstoke: Palgrave Macmillan, pp. 105–27.

Harding, M-L. (15 December 2005), 'Ham hits out at policy incoherence', *Health Service Journal*.

Jervis, P. and Plowden, W. (2003), *The Impact of Political Devolution on the UK's Health Services*, The Nuffield Trust, London

John, P.(1998), *Analysing Public Policy*, London.

Pinter Jones, K., Baggott, R. and Allsop, J. (2004), 'Influencing the National Policy Process: the Role of Health Consumer Groups', *Health Expectations*, **7**, pp. 18–28.

King's Fund (January 2002), *The Future of the NHS. A Framework for Debate*, King's Fund, London.

Larsen, Taylor-Gooby and Kananen (2006).'New Labour's Policy Style: A Mix of Policy Approaches', *Journal of Social Policy*, **35**(4), pp. 629–49.

Newman, J. (2001), *Modernising Governance. New Labour, Policy and Society*, Sage, London.

Parsons,W. (2001), 'Modernising Policy Making for the Twenty First Century: The Professional Model', *Public Policy and Administration*, **16**(3), pp. 93–110.

Pierre, J. and Peters, B.G. (2000), *Governance, Politics and the State*, St. Martin's Press, New York.

Quennell, P. (2001),'Getting their say, or getting their way? Has participation strengthened the patient "voice" in the National Institute for Clinical Excellence?' *Journal of Management in Medicine*, **15**(3) pp. 201–19.

Rhodes, RAW. (1997), *Understanding Governance. Policy Networks, Governance, Reflexivity and Accountability*, Open University Press, Buckingham

Richards, D. and Smith, M.J. (2002), *Governance and Public Policy in the UK*, Oxford University Press, Oxford

Smee, C. (2005), *Speaking Truth to Power: Two Decades of Analysis in the Department of Health*, The Nuffield Trust, London.

Chapter 5

Consumerism in Health Policy: Where Did it Come From and How Can it Work?

Ian Greener

Policy decisions position service users in particular roles through the assumptions they contain about their agency (Deacon & Mann, 1999; Greener, 2002a; Hoggett, 2001; Le Grand, 1997). At the extremes of this users can be located as sovereign 'queens', or fully-fledged consumers of welfare services, or instead as 'pawns', passive figures taking whatever services are offered to them (Le Grand, 2003). This paper examines how patients have been positioned through the choices available to them in the history of the National Health Service through an empirical examination of policy documents from 1944 through to 2000. It then goes onto explore the implications of these findings for our understanding of the history of consumerism in healthcare.

The paper presents a data-driven analysis of choice that closely dates the arrival of particular choices for patients, and therefore presents a finely grained chronology of how choices have changed the role that patients are meant to play in health services. Counter to much of the present literature on NHS policy, it suggests that choice is a relatively recent phenomena, so consumerism has entered health policy in a somewhat more subtle and cumulative way than is often assumed. Choice appears to have been used as means for achieving a particular policy goal – that of increasing the responsiveness of providers – but that responsiveness can be achieved through other means that position the users of health services in a way other than consumers, positions that are more viable and likely meet this goal.

Methods

The method for examining the policy documents here is based upon earlier work (Greener, 2003, 2004a, 2004b, 2005) that utilises a particular approach to textual analysis that addresses the difficult question faced in any discourse-related analysis of how to find a starting point for analysis in the text. Fairclough (2000), in his examination of the language of New Labour, counted words that appeared to frequently occur in the speeches of Prime Minister Tony Blair, and used these as the beginning of his approach. This paper finds it starting point instead through a more sophisticated approach. Policy documents concerned in broad terms with the organisation of health services in the UK (from 1944, 1946, 1962, 1968, 1970, 1971, 1972, 1983, 1989, 1996, 1997 and 2000) were converted into electronic form and processed as a single corpus of text. These documents comprise of inter-war proposals for the NHS (1944), the NHS Act (1946), the Porritt Report into health organisation – the only non-governmental report here, but used to represent the language of health in the Conservative governments of 1951–1964 in the absence of a significant organisational White Paper in that time; documents examining the first organisational reform of the NHS (1968, 1970, 1971, 1972), the 'Griffiths' management inquiry of 1983, the document outlining the Conservative internal market (1989), and the last White Paper produced by the Conservatives before losing power ('A Service with Ambitions, 1996); then, finally, Labour's first White Paper upon returning to power 'Modern, Dependable', 1997), and the NHS Plan (2000).

The corpus therefore has documents representing each governmental era, and is just short of 275,000 words, providing a rich source of data. The story of consumerism in healthcare beyond 2000 has taken another turn which I do not cover here because it would require in its own right (see new scholarship from Clarke et al., 2006; Greener, 2005), but I do consider the implications of our findings to 2000 for health policy generally beyond that date.

A computer software package, T-Lab, was used to examine each document in terms of the words which, relative to other documents but also relative to a general corpus of English usage, appeared to be either over-used or under-used through the calculation of the chi-squared statistic. These over and user-used words were then examined for words associated with various visions of consumerism (as in Aldridge, 2005; Gabriel & Lang, 2006; Paterson, 2006), with 'choice' in all its versions appearing overwhelmingly the most significant word (being amongst the most over-used words in 1946 and 1989 especially, and appearing nearly 300 times in the corpus so giving a rich variety of uses for analysis). Interestingly, words such as 'customer' or 'consumer', or any of their variants, scarcely ever appear in health policy documents, suggesting that policymakers are being extremely wary in using them.

Next usage of the word choice was examined to find other key words associated with it. The strongest co-association with choice (that is, the word most likely to appear with it) was 'independence', occurring 1/3 of the time. Independence is a goal of policy, suggesting that choice is meant to give service users more independence, but does not reveal very much about how health services should be organised to achieve this. Another key word co-associated with choice is 'patient', which is clearly a positioning of the user in health services, with one of the most important co-associations being 'responsive' and 'responsiveness' (a co-occurrence about 1/6 of the time across all the corpus, therefore being among the most statistically significant, but more importantly, substantively significant in terms of our study here).

These associations give a clear message, that there is a strong link between 'choice', and 'responsiveness' through 'patients' (which is confirmed by a more conventional analysis of the documents, see below) and that this relationship goes from choice to responsiveness but not necessarily in the opposite direction. In other words, responsiveness is usually the goal of increasing choice in health policy documents, but that responsiveness can also be achieved through other means. This insight is central to the message of the paper, and will be explored further below in the detailed data analysis.

Having selected the two key terms for examination in the document, choice (in all its versions) and 'responsiveness' (again in all its versions), all occurrences of those two words were extracted from the corpus (along with the paragraph either side within which they occurred) and thematically coded to find out who was being granted choices, over what, and for whom. In terms of responsiveness, coding was organised with a straightforward emphasis on finding out how responsiveness was meant to achieved, and what kind of responsiveness what being sought.

Passive Choices – Choice in the Setting Up of the NHS: 1944 and 1946

The first two documents analysed here are from the period of the NHS's creation. The 1944 text was the product of the inter-war coalition government, and the product of considerable negotiation, especially since the Beveridge Report of 1942 (Beveridge, 1942) that proposed a national health service for the post-war period (Powell, 1994). It proposed a health service that was far more evolutionarily related to service provision pre-war, not nationalising hospitals, and far more locally organised (Ministry of Health, 1944). By 1946, however, a Labour government was in place that was more overly Fabian (George & Wilding, 1994) than its predecessor, guided by Bevan and with nationalising hospital provision at its centre, abandoning the locally-based service favoured by Morrison which would have more closely resembled the 1944 Plan (Greener, 2006). As such, both documents are extremely concerned with the details of setting up the new health service, but certain key choices are highlighted that continue as themes in later years.

Central to the proposed health service in 1944 was the patient's right to choose his or her GP, but the relationship was conceptualised not in consumerist terms, but instead one based around a longer-term basis with the statement that 'public organisation must not destroy the sense of choice and personal association at the heart of "family doctoring"' ('General Practitioner Services'[1]) , implying that doctors were not to be picked up and abandoned as patients wished, but that the choice of GP was something to be entered into with gravity on both sides, it was an 'association'. The health centres proposed for the NHS would not alter this relationship, but did offer further examples of choice, with patients being free to choose a particular doctor in a health centre, or to choose a health centre and leave the specific details of the doctor unspecified. This was written at a time when single-GP surgeries were the dominant form, but clearly has resonance 60 years later when the public overwhelmingly belong to jointly managed practices and, despite being 'associated' with a particular GP, may never actually see that particular doctor.

In 1946 much discussion again surrounds the individual patient's choice of GP, with statements that lists of doctors within the NHS would be published, and that patients would choose who their practitioner from those lists. Patients were, unlike contemporary models of GP choice, not to be given any other information, but simply the list, and to register with a GP from it on that basis, suggesting they are

1 The use of an electronic corpus means that references to policy documents will be given in terms of either the name or the number of the nearest heading rather than the page number of the original document.

not required to behave in a particular discerning way. A second mention of choice is of interest, the specification that doctor will be able to choose which area they wish to practice in, giving choice rights to doctors as well as patients. This was the result of some negotiation with the state which wished to attempt to reallocate doctors into areas most in need (Klein, 2006).

In 1944 and 1946 patient choice of GP is not justified in terms of increased responsiveness. Instead the choice of GP was about association, a longer term and more professionally-oriented relationship. Instead there is a model of care that is organised around professional rather than consumer interests, in keeping with many existing accounts of the development of health organisation (Harrison & Pollitt 1994). Choice is present, but in a different context to the way we would view the term today, representing an informed choice by patients of doctors, and the right of doctors to choose to practice where they wished.

The Introduction of the Health Chooser – Choice and Responsiveness in Health Reform until 1989

There is then a remarkable period in which choice disappears from policy documents almost completely. The Porritt Report of 1962 (General Medical Services Committee, 1962) does not use either choice or responsiveness at all, being grounded in what Klein terms the age of 'technocratic change' (Klein, 2006) in which policymakers and other experts believed they could resolve health service problems through the rational use of planning techniques. This is largely continued in the first organisation reform of the NHS, and which resulted in a series of policy documents between 1968 and 1972 (Department of Health and Social Security, 1970, 1971; Ministry of Health, 1968; Secretary of State for Health and Social Services, 1972). The first three of these documents barely mention choice at all, and only then in terms of criteria by which health authorities and local authorities were to choose their members (demonstrating the dominance of planning again at this time). The final White Paper relating to the reorganisation of the NHS (1972), however, presents choice in two new ways, both of which were to mark the beginning of new conceptualisations of the user in health services.

First the government claimed it 'thinks it right for people to have an opportunity to exercise a personal choice to seek treatment privately' (section 23), breaking a long-held taboo of the mention of the health private sector, but also making clear that this was a consumer choice. Second, the document states that that 'The user….. to get the services best suited to his needs, his convenience and, as far as practicable, his choice' (section 48), giving a picture of an active healthcare agent capable of working between health and social care organisations to meet his or her needs, a theme to be followed up on in later years.

In the same period of reform, responsiveness begins to appear for the first time as a goal for health services. Responsiveness appeared in two senses, the first of which is cross-organisational. In 1970 it was suggested that 'if health services are to be made responsive to local and indeed individual needs, there must be closer involvement of members of health authorities in the running of health services' (section 20). This suggests that if health services are most closely linked to the organisation of health authorities then their responsiveness will be improved – a technocratic solution that does not necessarily involve more local participation but through the use of appointed officials. The second sense responsiveness appears argues for more decentralised services suggesting that the 'Government's proposals for integrated and decentralised services are designed to provide the flexibility for each local area to respond to change and adapt in services to meet it.' (section 109). This again suggests more local involvement, but again this was not to be achieved through the greater involvement of local people as either consumers or citizens, but through the involvement of their representatives in health authorities. This paved the way for the Community Health Council reforms of 1974 which were not about local democracy or consumerism, but instead through appointing individuals who would attempt to scrutinise local health decisions on behalf of the public.

As such, the first reorganisation of the NHS presents a view of health services that begins to expand patient choice (by making clear that the private sector represents a choice, and that choosing services implies crossing health and social care boundaries), and responsiveness (within a model of the expression of voice through appointed officials rather than through democratic means). There is the beginning of a consumerist discourse in terms of choice justified not through increased responsiveness, but instead apparently grounded in terms of offering potential exit from public provision for those able to pay. This is extremely worrying in terms of Hirschman's typology of exit, loyalty and voice (Hirschman, 1970) as it represents a case where what is likely to be the most articulate sector of society exits public provision for private, reducing the chance that poor services will result in complaint through voice, and subsequent change.

In 1979 the Thatcher government was elected promising to 'roll back the frontiers of the state' (Gamble, 1987), largely ignoring the Royal Commission into the NHS set up by their Labour predecessors, and expressing a more managerialist approach to reforming public services than their predecessors. This is expressed in their first policy document, 'Patients First' but the most significant policy document of the early 1980s was instead the NHS Management Inquiry organised by Roy Griffiths, and which reported in 1983. The 'Griffiths Report' marks the entry of general management into the NHS on the grounds of making health services more businesslike (Harrison et al., 1990).

Perhaps a little surprisingly, choice was not regarded as an important concept in the Griffiths report (Department of Health and Social Security, 1983) – it is not mentioned at all. This is because it was based not on a consumer-based NHS, but instead a customer-based one in which professionals were to be given responsibility for running health services. It was the role of managers to oversee this process, acknowledging that those running services might not necessarily to be managers by background, but could instead be doctors. Griffiths did not regard doctors in a naïve way, assuming that if they were set free from the state they would automatically deliver high quality care. Instead he made clear that, in order to manage, doctors had to be made accountable for their decisions in far more transparent ways, to understand their decisions carried resource implications, and that they were there to serve their localities. This is made clear in the reference responsiveness in the document, with the idea that the Community Health Councils (CHCs) could form a central part of managerial accountability by hospital managers responding to the information that they provided by formulating policies that would then form the basis of local performance measurement (section 13) This effectively means that CHCs would begin to become customers of the local hospital, moving us closer to consumerism, but given that CHCs were never representative of either patients or the public at large, still some distance from a consumerist model.

Extending Choice – Choice and Responsiveness in 1989 and 1996

By 1988 Thatcher believed that the NHS had become a 'bottomless financial pit' (Thatcher, 1993) and was in need of more significant reform. The resulting policy document, 'Working for Patients' (Secretary of State for Health, 1989) was the result of a long process of argument between Thatcher and Secretary of State Kenneth Clarke (Greener, 2002b; Timmins, 1995a, 1995b) in which the latter largely prevailed in putting in place reforms to introduce a 'quasi-market' into healthcare (Exworthy et al., 1999; Ferlie, 1994).

Choice makes a strong appearance in the 1989 document, appearing in a number of contexts. Following earlier examples patients are told they must be able to exercise a 'real choice between GPs (section 7.4), suggesting that this choice, which as was meant to be present according to documents as far back as 1944 and 1946, was not working quite as the architects of the NHS planned. This is perhaps because of doctors preventing patients from moving between practices, resulting in them being explicitly given the right in 1989 to be 'quite free to choose and change their doctor without any hindrance at all' (section 7.6). This is a far more consumerist notion than that of 1944 when the emphasis was on the association that comes from choosing a doctor, with no mention at all of changing that doctor, least of all 'without any hindrance'. This reconceptualises GPs and patients in a way that emphasises exit rather than association, implying that there is little different in the relationship than there is in any other market transaction. Instead of a GP service based on association and the expression of voice to deal with problems, this is clearly one based far more on the threat of exit (Hirschman, 1970).

A second theme following from earlier document was the re-emphasis on the role of the private sector in offering choices to patients. But again, this role had been extended by 1989. The private sector not only offered a choice for patients, but one that is actually good for the NHS. The document claims that that 'People who choose to buy health care outside the Health Service benefit the community by taking pressure off the Service and add to the diversity of provision and choice' (section 1.18). The role of the private sector as a provider to the NHS itself is also made clear, with the idea that 'introducing more choice into the provision of services will greatly increase the opportunities for managers to buy in services from the private sector where this will improve the services to patients' (section 9.12) This marks the beginning of the positioning of the private sector as a co-provider of health services into the NHS; since the beginning of the services history private medicine had worked alongside public through the contentious allowance of private beds inside public hospitals, but now these services were to be offered to NHS patients as well.

How was all this choice to work? Two questions appear – how is it to be financed, and who is meant to be making these new choices? The answer to the first is conceptually clearer than the second, but perhaps paradoxically, was to prove more difficult to achieve. Working for Patients is clear that 'Money must move with the patient so that hospitals which are efficient and effective, and attract more work, get the resources they need' (section 11.11), putting in place a system where choices count. Unfortunately, this was near impossible to achieve, with block contracting being about the closest the NHS came to attempting to allocate resources in line with patient demand at that time. As to who was meant to be making choices, the document is a little ambiguous, but appears to represent a principal-agent approach within which GPs , in consultation with patients, make choices on their behalf. The document states that 'Offering choice to patients means involving GPs far more in key decisions' (section 4.23) and 'General practice will play an even greater role in assisting patient choice and directing resources to match patient needs throughout the whole Health Service' (section 7.1). The choice process is a collaborative one in which GPs act on behalf of patients after discussing their care with them. Patient choice meant a greater involvement for patients in decisions, rather than making decisions for themselves.

In terms of what choices were meant to being made, again a range of possibilities appear from 'time or place of treatment' (section 1.12), a 'wider choice of meals' (section 1.13), and specific cases where location will be important, such long term care for the elderly. If patients weren't choosing their providers of care, they were to be offered additional consumer services once the care decisions had been made in collaboration with their doctor.

The 1989 White Paper also makes extensive use of 'responsiveness', and is the point where it clearly becomes a goal for health services. It appears in a number of contexts. First, there is the idea of responsiveness through decentralization (as in the 1970s reforms), in which by passing control over health services from the centre to more local levels, so 'to make the Health Service more responsive to the needs of patients, as much power and responsibility as possible will be delegated to local level' (section 1.8). But the White Paper took these ideas further, as the reforms' goals were explicitly specified as 'to extend patient choice, to delegate responsibility to those who are best placed to respond to patients' needs and wishes, and to secure the best value for money' (section 13.5). Responsiveness was to be achieved not by giving greater power to patients at this point, but instead by giving greater power to those that could respond to them - a principal-agent model because of its retention of the idea that clinicians had a role to play in directing patients through health services. This was clear in repeated suggestions that staff responsiveness would be key in improving health services with the claim that there would be 'greater satisfaction and rewards for those working in the NHS who successfully respond to local needs and preferences' (section 1.8).

So responsiveness in 1989 was about increasing patient choice initiative by staff treating patients as customers, but not consumers of health care. The difference between the two is that patients were not driving reforms through the suggestion that they knew better than clinicians what their needs were, but instead staff in health services were meant to interpret their needs through the use of their expertise, and to respond by giving the appropriate care.

By the middle of the 1990s, it appeared that health policy, from this highpoint of the advocacy of choice, had undergone something of a 'becalming' (Wainwright, 1998) and the furore over the introduction of the internal market had led to far less than it originally appeared.

The last White Paper of the Conservative era, published in 1996 (Secretary of State for Health, 1996), introduced two new uses of choice that were to built upon later. First, there was the use of choice as providing an example of how difficult it is for the government running the NHS; 'difficult choices about service and patient priorities sometimes have to be made' ('Setting priorities'). This was to be continued as a theme by Labour after 1997. Second, there was the idea that choices required the greater availability of information for patients, beginning to suggest that they might make choices more independently of their doctors. This meant that the co-production model of 1989 was gradually making way for one in which patients make choices for themselves. It was now the role of the NHS 'to provide information to patients and the public so they can make informed choices about their own lives, know what action to take to help themselves, know when and how to seek help, and so they can take part in decisions and choices about care and treatment' ('information') and People need good quality information…on how to stay healthy and choose healthy options' ('a well informed public). These examples suggest not only a more individual model of choice, but a broadening of the choice remit to include choice not only of treatment, but also of lifestyle – that as well as patient choice the NHS had a role to play in public health. Choice was a general health issue, following the publication of 'The Health of the Nation' in 1992 (Secretary of State for Health, 1992), a move toward the government accepting that the NHS needed to play a more active role in public health, but also suggesting that the public needed to ultimately take responsibility for making healthy decisions.

Responsiveness in 1996 had claims based around three ideas. First, in continuity with 1989, the idea it is staff that are central in responding the needs of patients, there is an acknowledgement that this was not just about clinical competence; 'The delivery of high-quality, responsive patient services relies not only on effective clinical skills but also on a wider range of competencies' ('A Highly Trained and Skilled Workforce'). Second, that responsiveness meant differing things in different contexts, suggesting the NHS needed to become more differentiated in its care to provide 'a responsive service sensitive to differing needs' ('Realising the ambition') but also to different circumstances between rural and urban locations. Third, there was the suggestion that patients were not only agents receiving care from professionals, but that they had a bigger role to play. The document claimed that the relationship between 'patients and professionals is changing' ('Professional development') and that the service was no longer about meeting patient needs, but instead represented 'the ambition of a high quality integrated service that is sensitive to the needs and wishes of patients' ('A responsive service'), moving us beyond patient needs to wishes, and towards a model of responsiveness that is more consumerist.

To Consumerism – Choice and Responsiveness under New Labour

By 1997, Labour had been returned to power, and quickly produced a new White Paper presenting their view of health organisation (Secretary of State for Health, 1997). Remarkably in terms of subsequent policy, there was no mention of patient choice at all – the White Paper instead suggested that the internal market experiment had failed on the grounds that it was wasteful and ineffective (section 1.22). The internal market however, was not abolished, however, despite Labour claims, with the purchaser provider split remaining in place, but in a different guise (Powell 1998). In terms of choice, the two main occurrences mentioned are in relation to 'tough choices facing the NHS' (section 1.24). The second mention moves us back to producer-led choices again, with a discussion of organisational choices. The document explores choices available to the new Primary Care Groups, but more significantly, how new budgeting arrangements will 'give GPs the maximum choice about the treatment option that suits individual patients' (section 9.8), which clearly suggested that it was GPs that made choices, but that they must do this on the individual level, finding the treatment that suits the particular patient before them. Labour then, did not appear to regard patient choice as central to their policy in 1997, with their organisational model becoming clearer through their usage of responsiveness.

If choices were few in 1997, there was a great deal more mention of responsiveness. First, there was the continued idea of making the best use of staff to achieve greater responsiveness so that such as nurses or doctors were 'best placed to understand their patients' needs as a whole and to identify ways of making local services more responsive'(section 2.7). This was taken further with the suggestion that organisational development techniques and that the 'NHS Executive will work with the health service locally to promote the organisational and personal development that must support clinicians and managers as they put these new arrangements in place and respond to the new challenges' (section 10.4).

Perhaps the most significant change present in the 1997 White Paper however, came in its continued movement closer to consumerism present in the statement that 'rising public expectations should be channelled into shaping services to make them more responsive to the needs and preferences of the people who use them' (section 3). This was close to the 1996 'needs and wishes', but took the idea even further in claiming that the public had a role not only in terms of having needs and preferences to be fulfilled, but that they also had expectations that could be utilised as a pressure for shaping health services. This was not professionals responding to needs, but instead professionals facing patients who had a clear idea of what service they wanted. Patients were moving beyond the customer model of 1989 in which the interpretation of their needs was the responsibility of doctors, to a position where doctors acted on their 'wishes' or 'preferences'– so being positioned as fully-formed consumers.

By 2000, and the release of the NHS Plan (Secretary of State for Health, 2000) this reference to health consumerism had becoming even more obvious. Patients 'have the right to choose a GP' (section 10.5), but following the 1996 approach, 'to make an informed choice of GP, a wider range of information about GP practices will be published' (section 10.5), linking choice of GP with available information.

Who was to make choices according to the NHS Plan? Once again, it appeared to be GPs rather than patients; 'Since 1999 the creation of primary care groups has restored choice of referrals to GPs' (section 10.7) and 'the choice GPs are able to exercise on behalf of their patients is important' (section 10.7). Where patients were to be given more choices was in the route through which they access the NHS; Patients 'are to be given more choice about accessing the NHS' (section 1.11), and 'patients to have choice emailing or phoning their practice for advice and booking appointments online' (section 1.11). This last idea suggested a movement towards a more flexible mode of health provision. If giving new care choices to patients was not central to New Labour's reform agenda in 2000, however, this quickly changed with a number of subsequent documents placing it as central to their idea of health reform (Department of Health, 2003, 2004, 2006; Minister of State for Department of Health et al., 2005; Secretary of State for Health, 2002).

As in 1989, choices appear about services after making care choices. Patients were to be given additional choices over hospital food as well as a new right, that of 'treatment at a time and hospital of the patient's choice' (section 10.20) in the situation where their operation had been cancelled and another binding date could not be offered within 28 days. This is a hark back to another Conservative policy of the 1980s and 1990s, the Citizens' Charter, which attempted to introduce a series of clearly specified rights for care that would allow patients to know more clearly that standards of service they could expect (Department of Health, 1991). In many respects Labour's health policy can be regarded as a series of responses to previous policy initiatives, but they are all based around a particular language – that of consumerism as a means to drive up responsiveness.

Responsiveness is as central to the 2000 document as it was in 1989, but went further. In terms of staff responsiveness it is a matter not just for the development of skills for clinicians and managers when in-post, instead it is now far more central so that 'there will be reforms to the health curricula to give everyone working in the NHS the skills and knowledge to respond effectively to the individual needs of patients' (section 9.18). The idea of responding to the 'individual' is present everywhere, 'today successful services thrive on their ability to respond to the individual needs of their customers' (section 2.12) – a statement that would have been unthinkable in a health policy document even twenty years before, and this is further emphasised by making clear that 'the NHS must also be responsive to the different needs of different populations in the devolved nations and throughout the regions and localities' (section 4), continuing with the theme of responding to difference present in other documents. A new context for responsiveness appeared around patient complaints where 'the government will act to reform the complaints procedure to make it more independent and responsive to patients' (section 10.21), giving the newly created health consumers not only the right to be heard in their interactions with health professionals, but a reassertion of the right to complain if they felt their voice was not being taken enough into account.

Discussion and Conclusions

The analysis of policy documents in this way suggests a number of conclusions.

First, that choice agendas are not inextricably associated with competition-based reforms, but often come to be linked with them as the means by which health services are meant to become more responsive. Instead, there is an alternative history of policy based around health service responsiveness that has little to do with choice agendas, but instead is based around attempting to make staff more responsive to patients through other means. Choice and responsiveness come to be closely associated at particular moments of health service reform (1989 being an obvious example), but choice does not automatically lead to competition (as in the patients choice of GP), and responsiveness can be achieved through other methods than offering patients greater choice. There is clearly a link between choice (through exit) and voice, but it is, as Hirschman suggested, rather more complicated than a relationship of substitution (Hirschman, 1970). Offering exit may be neither appropriate nor possible, and fostering responsiveness through voice may yet prove to be a more viable alternative.

Second, the evidence suggests that choice in the NHS is not new, that in fact it has been present in health policy documents since before the creation of the NHS. Health services in the UK have always been based on the principle that individuals have the right to choose their own GP, and the right to choose private healthcare. What has changed is the nature of the relationship patients have with their general practitioner and which has moved from being an 'association' to one in which it is easy to change doctor or change practice in today's NHS. In Hirschman's terms, a situation of wishing to negotiate care through a process of voice, and an association of loyalty to public services, has changed one instead where only exit is advocated (Minister of State for Department of Health et al., 2005). When combined with a reform agenda that places individual patient choice at its centre, this creates a model where patients, positioned as consumers, can make demands upon GPs with the threat of exit, and where they do not receive what they want, keep moving until they find a doctor amenable to their requirements. This is not to advocate a return to the days where patients found it impossible to change GPs, or where GPs were able to ignore patients' needs. However, treating GPs as service providers that can be dismissed at will goes against the ideas of 'family doctoring' upon which the UK health system was founded, and asks questions as whether this is really necessary or desirable.

Third, claims that consumerism have become central to the NHS can be justified in terms of the way that policy has positioned and described the role of patients, but that the process through which patients have become repositioned as consumers has been far more incremental than is often presented – health policy did not undergo a big bang, in which suddenly patients acquired new rights, but rather this has been a long and drawn out process where a rather slower evolution has occurred. By the 1970s there is a discourse around achieving greater responsiveness through decentralisation emerging as well as the founding of the CHCs which, whilst hardly positioning patients as consumers, did provide a means for attempting to provide greater local service accountability in a similar way to organisations such as the citizens' advice bureau. This discourse of decentralization continues into the 1980s through the 'Griffiths reforms', until 'Working for Patients' in which patients are positioned at customers, with their needs being interpreted through health professionals and being met that way. After this, there is a gradual further move to health consumerism, with health professionals being urged not just to respond to needs, but also patient 'wishes', an acknowledgement that rising patient expectations can be used as a driver of health reform.

The birth of the health consumerism has been a long one and confused one. This is because it is not always clear exactly who is meant to be making choices for patients. In 1989 it is usually GPs, but often GPs and patients together. By 2000 it is usually still GPs, but this seems to have been abandoned in policy since that time which suggests that patients, largely unaided, will be choosing both the location and time of their treatment, which again moves us towards the health consumerism which often appears increasingly advocated in later policy documents. In subsequent reforms it has become clearer that it is patients that are meant to making choices in healthcare, but not exactly how these choices are meant to be made.

A fourth claim is that that the slow evolution of responsiveness and choice allows us to see different models of health consumerism and its link to responsiveness, and this allows us to assess the viability of each. In the 1970s responsiveness was pursued through the greater involvement of health authority members, a model based very much on local accountability through council operations. By the 1980s this democratic element appears to largely disappear, but is reinstated in 1997 when 'responsive' and 'accountable' frequently appear together , although the means by which this is mean to be achieved are often unclear. However, there is clearly a link between responsiveness and local accountability that is a coherent approach to reform, and an alternative to the idea that responsiveness can only come from market-based reforms.

A model of health reform in which choice drives responsiveness carries with it the implication (although it seldom appears in policy documents) that competition will be the means for this. This has two variants; the 1989 version in which GPs act on behalf of patients, and the new model, post-2000, in which fully formed health consumers make the choices either with their doctors or through their doctors. Responsiveness is therefore achieved by the threat of patient exit to another GP, where the patient is not given what he or she wants, or through the choice the patient makes not being up to scratch, in which case complaint as well as exit will probably occur. This appears to be the dominant model of choice and responsiveness in present reforms, but asks rather a lot of patients in asking them to choose between health services where both little or no information exists, but also presumes that patients actually want these choices, when there is very little evidence to suggest that they do (Fotaki et al., 2005). The 1989 model, in which GPs refer in consultation with patients, is perhaps more plausible, and it also seems sensible that health services need to become more responsive to issues such as waiting and the preservation of patient dignity than they have been in the past. However, choice and exit are not necessary for either of these goals - instead the recent refocusing on complaint offers the potential for patients to engage in voice rather than exit, and so improve services not just for themselves but also for others. Voice may be more viable long-term as a means of securing responsiveness than choice, and the use of patient complaint is vital means for securing this, provided that managers can focus on ensuring that complaints are investigated independently and quickly.

As to what has driven the movement towards health consumerism, there seem to be two possibilities. First, is the version present in policy documents, that consumerism has arisen as a result of the lack of responsiveness in the past, with patients having had to wait too long, with wards not being clean enough, and with medical records often going missing, and because of these problems, and the rise in consumer expectations generally, the present is not good enough. There is clearly an element of truth in this – health organisations have often been careless in their dealing with patients. But the second explanation, that health consumerism has been deliberately 'stoked up' through Secretaries of State continually raising the expectations of patients in health policy documents and speeches, also bears some scrutiny (Clarke et al., 2006). The view of patients as consumers often describes a view of the world entirely foreign to patients or professionals within health services, and which is based on assumptions about health organisation that, as I have suggested above, may be neither viable nor what patients want (Newman & Vidler, 2006). It often appears as if policymakers, by positioning patients as consumers, are hoping to achieve a legitimacy for reforms by speaking for the 'people', that cannot be achieved in the implementation of those policies.

A final conclusion is that it is noticeable that choice increasingly has another dimension to it – that of patients taking personal responsibility for health choices. This is the 'new public health', in which government increasingly seeks to pass the responsibility not only of making choices for the time and place of treatment to individuals, but also makes it clearer that patients are responsible for the choices in their everyday life (Peterson & Lupton, 1996). The often hidden side of health consumerism is that patients are positioned not only as choosers of treatment, but also as choosers of lifestyle, and that they must take greater responsibility for making healthy choices of food and exercise. This is clearly a significant move; for much of its history the NHS has focused on the provision of treatment for illness rather than the education of the public to be healthy. Health consumerism, however gives patients the right to demand what they wish from health services, but also greater responsibility for what they wish for. If patient choice is taken to one extreme, patients could request treatments that have unproven efficacy, but to have to take the responsibility for making those choices. At the same time, choices about lifestyle and exercise taken over a number of years can have profound implications for an individual's health that might not be apparent whilst the person is, for example, drinking heavily and smoking. If the state is warning individuals that such behaviour is likely to damage health, and the language of 'touch choices' facing health services in the future is also becoming increasingly prevalent, it may be that the NHS will increasingly refuse to act as a safety net in future years, as health services might become increasingly be prioritised.

Acknowledgements

Thanks to John Clarke and Richard Simmons for their comments on an earlier version of this paper which was published by the ESRC as a working paper as a part of its 'Cultures of Consumption' Programme which helped fund the research that went into the writing of this chapter.

References

Aldridge, A. (2005), *The Market*, Polity Press, Cambridge.

Beveridge, W. (1942), *Social Insurance and Allied Services*, HMSO, London.

Clarke, J., Smith, N., Vidler, E. (2006), 'The Indeterminacy of Choice: Political, Policy and Organisational Implications', *Social Policy and Society*, **5**, 327–36.

Deacon, A., Mann, K. (1999), 'Agency, Modernity and Social Policy', *Journal of Social Policy*, **28**, 413–35.

Department of Health (1991), *The Patient's Charter*, London.

Department of Health (2003), *Building on the Best: Choice, Responsiveness and Equity in the NHS*, London.

Department of Health (2004), *Choosing Health: Making healthy Choices Easier*, London.

Department of Health (2006), *Patient Choice becomes a Reality across the NHS*, London.

Department of Health and Social Security (1970), *National Health Service: The Future Structure of the National Health Service*, HMSO, London.

Department of Health and Social Security (1971), *National Health Service Reorganisation: Consultative Document*, HMSO, London.

Department of Health and Social Security (1983), *NHS Management Inquiry*, HMSO, London.

Exworthy, M., Powell, M., Mohan, J. (1999), 'The NHS: Quasi-market, quasi-hierarchy or quasi-network?' *Public Money and Management*, **19**, 15–22.

Fairclough, N. (2000), *New Labour, New Language?*, Routledge, London.

Ferlie, E. (1994), 'The Creation and Evolustion of Quasi Markets in the Public Sector: early evidence from the National Health Service', *Policy and Politics*, **22**, 105–12.

Fotaki M., Boyd A., Smith L., McDonald R., Roland M., et al. (2005), *Patient Choice and the Organization and Delivery of Health Services: Scoping Review*, NCCSDO, London.

Gabriel, Y. and Lang, T. (2006), *The Unmanageable Consumer*, Sage, London.

Gamble, A. (1987), *The Free Economy and the Strong State*, Macmillan, London.

General Medical Services Committee (1962), *A Review of the Medical Services of Great Britain: Report of the Medical Services Review Committee*, Social Assay, London.

George, V. and Wilding, P. (1994), *Ideology and Social Welfare*, Harvester Wheatsheaf, London.

Greener, I. (2002a), 'Agency, social theory and social policy', *Critical Social Policy*, **22**, 688–706.

Greener, I. (2002b), 'Understanding NHS Reform: The Policy-Transfer, Social Learning, and Path-Dependency Perspectives', *Governance*, **15**, 161–84.

Greener, I. (2003), 'Who Choosing What?: The evolution of 'choice' in the NHS, and its implications for New Labour', in C. Bochel, N. Ellison, M. Powell (eds) *Social Policy Review*, **15**, 49–68, Policy Press, Bristol.

Greener, I. (2004a), 'Changing Words, Changing Times: What difference has the change in Health Secretary made?', *British Journal of Health Care Management*, **10**, 86–8.

Greener, I. (2004b), 'The Three Moments of New Labour's Health Policy Discourse', *Policy and Politics*, **32**, 303–16.

Greener, I. (2005), 'The Role of the Patient in Healthcare Reform: Customer, Consumer or Creator?', in S. Dawson, C. Sausmann (eds) *Future health organisations and systems*, 227–45, Palgrave, Basingstoke.

Greener, I. (2006), 'Path Dependency and the Creation and Reform of the NHS', in N. Smyth (ed.) *Health Care in Transition*, **3**, Nova Science, New York.

Harrison, S., Hunter, D., Pollitt, C. (1990), *The Dynamics of British Health Policy*, Unwin Hyman, London.

Harrison, S., Pollitt, C. (1994), *Controlling Health Professionals: The Future of Work and Organization in the National Health Service*, Open University Press, Buckingham.

Hirschman, A. (1970), *Exit, Voice and Loyalty: Responses to Decline in Firms, Organizations and States*, Harvard University Press, London.

Hoggett, P. (2001), 'Agency, Rationality and Social Policy', *Journal of Social Policy*, **30**, 37–56.

Klein, R. (2006), *The New Politics of the NHS: From creation to reinvention*, Radcliffe Publishing, Abingdon.

Le Grand, J. (1997), Knights, Knaves or Pawns? Human Behaviour and Social Policy, *Journal of Social Policy*, **26**, 149–69.

Le Grand, J. (2003), *Motivation, Agency and Public Policy: Of Knights, Knaves, Pawns and Queens*, Oxford University Press, Oxford.

Minister of State for Department of Health, Minister of State for Local and Regional Government, Minister of State for School Standards (2005), 'The Case for User Choice in Public Services', Public Administration Select Committee into Choice, Voice and Public Services, London.

Ministry of Health (1944), *A National Health Service*, HMSO, London,

Ministry of Health (1968), *National Health Service: The Administrative Structure of the Medical and Related Services in England and Wales*, HMSO, London.

Newman, J., Vidler, E. (2006), Discriminating Customers, Responsible Patients, Empowered Users: Consumerism and the Modernisation of Health Care, *Journal of Social Policy*, **35**, 193–209.

Paterson, M. (2006), *Consumption and Everyday Life*, Taylor and Francis, London.

Peterson, A. and Lupton, D. (1996), *The New Public Health: Health and Self in the Age of Risk*, Sage, London.

Powell, M. (1994), The Forgotten Anniversary? An Examination of the 1944 White Paper, *Social Policy and Administration*, **28**, 337.

Powell, M. (1998), 'New Labour and the "new" UK NHS', *Critical Public Health*, **8**, 167–73.

Secretary of State for Health (1989), *Working for Patients*, HMSO, London.

Secretary of State for Health (1992), *The Health of the Nation: A Strategy for Health in England*, HMSO, London.

Secretary of State for Health (1996), *The NHS: A Service with Ambitions*, HMSO, London.

Secretary of State for Health (1997), *The New NHS: Modern, Dependable*, HMSO, London.

Secretary of State for Health (2000), *The NHS Plan: A Plan for Investment, A Plan for Reform*, HMSO, London.

Secretary of State for Health (2002), *Delivering the NHS Plan: Next Steps on Investment and Reform*, HMSO, London.

Secretary of State for Health and Social Services (1972), *The National Health Service Reorganisation: England*, HMSO, London.

Thatcher, M. (1993), *The Downing Street Years*, Harper Collins, London.

Timmins, N. (1995a), *The Five Giants*, Fontana, London.

Timmins, N. (1995b), 'How three top managers nearly sank the reforms', *Health Service Journal*, 11–3.

Wainwright, D. (1998), 'Disenchantment, Ambivalence and the Precautionary Principle: The Becalming of British Health Policy', *International Journal of Health Services*, **28**, 407–26.

Chapter 6

Choice, Voice and the Structures of Accountability in the New NHS

Susan Pickard

This chapter looks at user responsiveness in the 'new' NHS after 1997. To do so, it applies Hirschman's (1970) framework of 'exit' and 'voice' both to health policy and to the mechanisms set up by such policy, drawing from two separate studies carried out at NPCRDC, University of Manchester between 2000 and 2004 and in both of which the author was involved. These studies examined firstly the governance arrangements of nine Primary Care Trusts (PCTs) and their relationship to user responsiveness, modernisation and accountability, (e.g. Sheaff et al., 2004) and secondly involved a further 12 PCTs in a focus on clinical governance processes including the role of users in setting and monitoring such processes (Pickard, Sheaff and Dowling, 2006).

We begin by setting out Hirschman's 'exit and voice' framework. We then set the context for this examination by briefly tracing the different notions of accountability to users of the NHS and others before and after 1997. Next, it analyses the effectiveness of the feedback mechanisms established by the 'new' NHS and operating within the different governance structures of hierarchies, quasi-markets and networks in primary care organisations . In each instance it links this with the nature of the accountabilities present within each type of governance structure. We conclude by relating this back to Hirschman's original theory and drawing out some implications for improving user responsiveness within the NHS.

Hirschman's Theory of 'Exit and Voice'

Hirschman's analysis contrasts exit and voice as two 'recovery' mechanisms for making organisations responsive to their users. Exit is usually found in competitive business enterprises and is associated with economic markets and voice in public bodies or democratically responsive organisations. Neither method, says Hirschman, singly or in combination, is better necessarily than any other: it all depends on the sensitivity of the organisation to whatever method is in place. Hirschman's theory remains very relevant today as voice and exit are used in varying combinations in different health systems internationally to improve the responsiveness to users. However, since Hirschman's theory first appeared, however, two trends have complicated the equation between exit and markets and voice and politically accountable bodies. Firstly, health care quasi-markets have appeared in many countries, frequently containing both voice and exit mechanism; secondly networks have appeared as governance structures or, increasingly, 'quasi-networks' since 1997 (Exworthy et al., 1999).

Pre-1997: Accountability within a Neo-liberal Paradigm

During the 1980s and 1990s the public administration paradigm and associated accountability was replaced by a neo-liberal paradigm emphasising managerial (upwards) and consumer (downwards) accountability in healthcare within a new public management (Hood, 1995) based on a differing conception of principal and agent motivation (Le Grand, 2003). As managerial control tightened, quasi-markets were correspondingly to be the means of making the system responsive to purchasers, in the sense of both commissioners and patients while non-legally enforceable contracts were the primary means for ensuring accountability of both a fiduciary and quality nature (Flynn et al., 1996).

As far as professionals were concerned, the Griffiths Inquiry changed the medical dominance in principle at least by introducing general managers, various budgets performance indicators and medical management roles. However the medical profession continued to elude the grasp of upwards accountability and threats to their autonomy (Harrison and Ahmad, 2000). Doctors remained accountable for their clinical performance only to their professional bodies and the holding of managerial roles such as clinical directorships may have actually increased their power. Medical audit remained a strictly professional concern and the links between the findings of external monitoring organizations such as the Audit Commission and the Clinical Standards Advisory Group and the possibility of sanctions remained weak. GP fund holders (GPFHs), while being accountable for their financial management, remained unaccountable for the clinical services they provided with their fund holding budgets (Harrison and Dixon, 2000) with self-regulation for professionals remaining during this time the 'principle of essence' (Stacey, 1992: 215).

Meanwhile, looking downwards, the Conservative government's focus was a consumerist one, on tax payer as customer, which was often contrasted with the citizenship approach and the latter's emphasis instead on the rights of citizens within a democratic society. However, the two philosophies were not considered contradictory in the eyes of the Conservatives: on the contrary they saw market-based responsiveness as a more tangible, direct form of accountability to the individual than the diffuse workings of a distant representative government system could ever be and transformed him/her from the hapless and impotent welfare client, associated with the public administration paradigm, and into the 'heroic' consumer (Rouse and Smith, 1999).

Another way in which the two philosophical approaches towards choice could be contrasted was in terms of the mechanisms they employed. The consumerist approach was linked with mechanisms that were largely responsive in nature: apart from exit, there were the weaker expressions of 'voice' such as satisfaction questionnaires, complaints procedures, consumer audit and the Patient's Charter. Although exit from GPFHs happened rarely, the threat of it occurring was an important restraint on

GPFHs behaviour (Le Grand, 2003). The citizenship approach, on the other hand, made use of structural mechanisms, built into organizations, and which could act on behalf of wider groups than specific consumer groups and think strategically. Mechanisms included joint consultative and joint planning committees feeding into decision making within health authorities and Community Health Councils (CHCs) separate from Health Authorities (HAs) but funded by the Department of Health (DH). In addition Health Panels, Local Voices and Citizens' Juries convened for specific purposes. Membership, however, was 'captive' and could not move elsewhere.

Consumer choice in the quasi-market established by the same Conservative government in health did not occur as predicted, however, and there was little evidence of real choice on either an individual or collective basis during this time. The main concern of providers was the purchaser, not the individual user, who acted on behalf of large groups of users in a proxy form, either as GPs or commissioners. Restrictions on involving local users included difficulties in specifying outcomes in contracts, uncertainty about how to build 'local voice' information into purchasing plans, the continuation of inflexible block contracts and the fact that health care organisations remained virtual monopolies (Flynn et al., 1996). The proliferation of a 'new magistracy' (Stewart, 1995) and a hollowed-out state in which a multiplication of non-accountable multi-level governance replaced centralised governance structures (Rhodes, 1997) contributed towards producing a 'democratic deficit' during this time. When New Labour was voted in, it was with passionate declarations of intent to strengthen user choice in the UK within the context of a responsive democracy.

Accountability in the Third Way Paradigm

'New' Labour officially abolished the internal market straight after it was elected in 1997 but it retained the purchaser/provider split while placing the emphasis on co-operative and collaborative relationships between all stakeholders, including patients and citizens. The latter were to be at the very heart of decision-making henceforth. The NHS was from now on to be an institution that is 'accountable to patients, open to the public and shaped by their views' (DH, 1997: 2.4). PCTs, the main drivers in a newly crafted primary-care led NHS, were to involve their 'local community' which meant local government, patients and citizens and voluntary organisations where appropriate. The aim was to help restore confidence in and hence legitimacy of the NHS, ensure improved outcomes for individual patients, more appropriate user of health services at local level and potentially greater cost effectiveness of services (NHSE, 1998).

However, managerial accountability was strengthened even more under New Labour through such mechanisms as performance indicators, league tables and the extensive use of audit. At national level, 'inspection, incentives, information and intervention, operating under the umbrella of clear national standards will help reshape services' (Secretary of State for Health, 2000: 30) and the government held PCTs accountable for meeting over 40 publically acknowledged mandatory 'targets'.

While primary care was henceforth to be in the driving seat, a new kind of upwards accountability was imposed upon the medical profession. 'A First Class Service' (DH, 1998), which introduced the concept of clinical governance, was the first attempt to bring clinical activity within the same managerial framework as that applying to the rest of the NHS. Clinical governance has been called 'the most systematic strategy for controlling doctors ever attempted in the NHS' (Harrison and Dowswell, 2000: 93) and operated through the National Institute for Clinical Excellence (NICE), through 'National Service Frameworks' (NSFs) and through the Commission for Health Improvement (CHI) all of which instituted a central control on what had formerly been individual clinical autonomy.

Medical accountability downwards, however, received no such precise attention and coupled with that was a notable lack of experience of primary care in engaging with patients in any way whatsoever beyond the consulting room. Those practices that had involved users in planning or decision-making before 1997 were exceptional (Colin-Thome, 1996; Robinson, 1996) and the Audit Commission found a poor record of involving the public even among the more innovative "first-wave" fund holders (Audit Commission, 1996) despite the responsibility on them set out in the Accountability Framework for GP fund holding for them to be accountable to patients and the wider public.

Thus from the outset several political objectives or tendencies threatened to clash and possibly obstruct public choice and involvement. A centralist agenda was meant to co-exist with local drivers and there seemed a similar incompatibility between upward and downward accountabilities. Much would depend on the nature of the precise accountabilities built into the differing governance structures found in PCTs and their ability to facilitate public choice. It is to these we turn next.

New NHS Policy: Possibilities of Exit and Voice?

NHS policies for promoting user responsiveness emphasise democratic accountability, rights of citizenship, partnership, empowerment and choice and changing PCTs' organisational culture accordingly (DH, 2000, 2001, 2003, 2004).

For communicating users' demands to NHS decision-makers at both national and local levels, policy documents recommend consultation, collaboration and the use of networks and consumer research. They also recommend involving users directly in NHS decision-making including; citizens' juries, community development; and local government scrutiny. The central mechanism is inclusion of lay non-executive directors (NEDs) on PCT Boards, one of whom is expressly designated 'lay representative'.

All mechanisms set up by policy concern voice not exit, eight existing at the organisational level and three at the individual patient level. One exit- based policy includes the right to choose one's individual GP but there is little emphasis placed upon this and the Patient Prospectuses which PCTs have published since 2002 give information on how to access local NHS services but not how to compare them (Noble et al., 2005).

While NHS services are accountable clinically and managerially to PCTs, the latter do not directly manage most NHS services for their local populations but arrange these services through a variety of Trusts, GPs, voluntary and other providers. It is through NHS governance structures that PCTs hold these agencies accountable through a combination of hierarchical, quasi-market and network governance structures (Flynn et al., 1996; Dowling et al., 2003). Not that governance structures should be seen as merely mechanisms for accountability: they 'involve accountability but are equally structures of policy development and policy implementation' (Mulgan, 2000: 565). We turn next to an examination of the user responsiveness found in each governance type within PCTs.

User Responsiveness Mechanisms through Hierarchical Governance

Hierarchical governance structures exist both within PCTs and between a PCT and the higher level NHS bodies (Strategic Health Authority (SHA), DH) who manage it. Within PCTs, managerial authority rests with a Board of Directors consisting mainly of public appointees but with minority medical representation and a Professional Executive Committee, consisting mainly of GPs but with a minority of members from other professions and NHS management. Through the Chief Executive the Board line-manages the directly-employed PCT staff (nurses and a minority of PMS salaried doctors). All inputs and working processes are open in this environment to an employer's scrutiny through management information systems and non-compliance with directives can be met by financial penalties, dismissal and coercion (Dowling et al., 2004).

Hierarchical mechanisms classically employ 'voice' as the instrument of user choice but our fieldwork discovered these to be functioning at a low level. We found the influence of user voice on planning and service changes to be largely intangible. There seem to be four main reasons for this. Firstly, the main role for effecting user involvement in the PCT, that of the non-executive director (NED) is ill-defined and lacking in authority. Secondly, national priorities which are compulsory overwhelm local priorities, generated by user involvement. Thirdly, user involvement has proved challenging for PCTs. Fourthly, approaches to involving the local community in PCT decision-making were neither well-developed or widely utilised and almost no use was made of consumer research.

As noted, the main voice mechanism within PCT hierarchies was through the appointment of lay NEDs but generally that mechanism was weak. Generally NEDs were active but not powerful and their role was procedural but vague. As one lay representative said about his role:

> I would see it more about influence ... about unblocking blockages ... or ... contributing a different discussion and dimension to the thinking.

In some PCTs, lay reps had to struggle to put anything on the agenda themselves and in some cases this did not in fact prove possible. In any case, this and other studies (Pickard et al., 2001) have found that NEDs in PCTs have been perceived (by themselves and others within the PCT) as having less influence than either professionals or managers and sometimes their role is perceived to be to legitimate decisions in reality made by others. In the words of one NED: 'I ... said at the Board meeting last week I was beginning to look like a rubber stamp' (Lay rep, PCT 4).

Certainly, local issues came lower in priority than national, centrally-driven directives. As one NED described:

> We find it less easy to involve people in real decisions because a lot of the things, by the time they've made their way to PCTs, the decisions are made, we're just implementing them so we might consult people on the implementation of something rather than on whether or not we should do it (Executive Director (of Modernisation), PCT 5).

Because of the pre-eminence of national targets, as another lay rep commented,

> that takes away a huge amount of scope from the Board for making the sorts of decisions that I would have wanted to take.

Beyond the Board's management team, approaches to involving the wider public or local community were not well-developed or utilised during the years of our research. Engagement with the wider public even in the larger PCTs was rudimentary or non-existent with the PCTs 'still debating the nature of public involvement' (lay rep, PCT 4). There was also a widespread consensus among our respondents that the mechanisms for user responsiveness were flawed: the Patient Advice and Liaison Service (PALs) were considered by some to be ill-suited to primary care, for example:

> You have this nice person in the hospital reception who helps you find your way around and get to wherever you want to go, and smooth out all the problems. That model simply doesn't translate to primary care where we have dozens of different entry points' (PCT chair, site 2).

Equally poorly developed voice mechanisms were noted across the whole of the NHS. Buckland and Gorin (2001) found there to be limited consumer involvement in the NHS R&D Regional Programmes and the Commission for Health Improvement (CHI) had not found any examples of excellence in voice mechanisms for the public in any of the NHS organisations it reviewed to 2003 (Gilbert, 2003).

These tensions and conflicting priorities were reflected in the nature of the accountabilities perceived by PCTs to be overwhelmingly upwards in nature. Informants, particularly chief executives and board chairs, described their chief accountability being that to the Strategic Health Authority (SHA), the Department of Health and Secretary of State. One SHA informant stated that if main targets were breached "the effect is the removal of the chief executive" (SHA rep, site 7); the chair could also be removed (Dowling et al., 2004). By comparison, the PCT interviewees said they considered themselves accountable to the general public 'informally'. One deputy chief executive explained that local responsiveness was constrained by the 'pretty comprehensive' requirements of the NHS Plan and said:

> If you do stuff that's not in the NHS Plan questions will be asked saying: 'Why are you doing them?' (Deputy CE, site 3).

User Responsiveness through Quasi-market Governance

PCTS commission providers in three quasi-markets: for acute and specialised mental hospital services, through service level agreements(SLAs), which replaced the old 'contracts' after 1997; for a large minority of general practices through local ('PMS') contracts; and for private primary care services, most often paramedical care and nursing homes. Each PCT is sole commissioner for its resident population who have no exit to another NHS commissioner. Commissioners, meanwhile, have the choice of exit or non-payment of an unsatisfactory provider. User exit was limited to general practice level.

Information transfers are stipulated by service level agreements (or contracts) and by relationality (Dowling et al., 2004) Exit was only used by PCTs in a tiny minority of cases among our sample – in only one case, in fact (from a small private provider of physiotherapy). In any case SLAs between providers and purchasers were so weakly defined that commissioners themselves found it impossible to influence them directly and the possibility of user views impacting them was almost non-existent. Nor did PCTs monitor user exit from general practices as a means to making the latter more user-responsive. In any case, this was not a practical option for many individuals: three sites had unfilled GP vacancies and so there was little option in reality – exit could mean losing GP access altogether. The vagueness of SLAs meant that they were not really amenable to users' influence or, in many cases, to PCT influence either. They continue a story that began under the market-type orientation of the NHS that existed till 1997, when commissioners in the NHS quasi-market did little to make NHS Trusts more accountable to them (Flynn et al., 1996). This was particularly the case for mental health services, despite the fact that several of the PCTs also formed networks with neighbouring PCTs for jointly commissioning mental health services which gave them administrative economies of scale and, it would have been reasonable to assume, should have increased their bargaining weight. However, as one Mental Health Lead (MHL) said:

> We (PCT) don't seem to be able to get to the bottom of exactly how much ... they've got and what they've done with it (MHL, site 3).

User Responsiveness through Networked Governance

PCTs rely on network forms of governance most significantly in their relationship with GPs. In each PCT a PEC co-ordinated a local network of all GPs, mediating their relationship with the PCT Board. These networks were the main link between PCTs and general practices and were constructed mainly around clinical governance. They were elected or nominated by local GPs with only one exception in our study sites, where the PCT recruited PEC members by formal interview.

In general, information in networks is to some extent volunteered by network members which relies heavily on intra-network communication systems (Dowling et al., 2004) and within the GP networks that we observed persuasion, knowledge management and 'soft coercion' were the means by which PCTs could influence

GPs. There were no means of 'bringing to heel' those GPs who chose not to comply with the clinical governance agenda (Sheaff et al., 2004). There was no difference in this respect between GPs, whether salaried or GMS.

Within these networks neither voice nor exit would appear to offer obvious tools for choice: instead 'culture change', in terms of changing GP attitudes, is the main medium by which PCTs can promote lay influence. However, we found little evidence that this had occurred in any sense (Pickard et al., 2002). At Board level, lay members were not involved in clinical governance priority setting at the time of our study. Beyond Board level, we found scattered evidence of involvement of patients in clinical governance discussions at GP practice level but it was sparse and uneven and focused on discrete services such as teenage pregnancy. In the two clinical specialties on which we focused – mental health and coronary heart disease – we found very few examples of user involvement.

Networks with local government seem to be most significant of all network types in effecting user involvement and there were some examples of voice-associated activities occurring within Local Strategic Partnerships, for example with consultations for out -of -hours services taking place before any formal consultation has begun. Nevertheless, within primary care, our GP informants viewed the cycle of influence as operating in a somewhat reverse direction from that intended by the PCT Board. Instead of the PEC and GP networks being a conduit by which the Board's responses to user demands were transmitted to general practices, these informants argued that patient opinions were transmitted via GPs to the PEC and thence to the PCT Board. The PEC chair of PCT 1 felt that the PEC were involved in responding to users anyway because 'most of them are working with service users every day'. This comment indicates that culture change, if it is indeed occurring, includes many GPs lagging well behind.

These examples illustrate the weak responsiveness of networks and the soft accountability associated with them, particularly within GP networks. PEC chairs and other GP members played down the extent to which GPs were accountable to the PCT. Comments were: "GPs are only accountable to the GMC (General Medical Council)"; "GPs can do what they like within their contract." This applied both to PMS and GMS doctors, surprisingly: one of our salaried GP informants thought her PCT held her even less accountable than the independent GPs because the PCT regarded its salaried GPs as a minor exception and, in addition, being short of GPs, it did not want to antagonise her with 'differential treatment'. One Chair suggested the PMS 'doesn't make, alter the basic nature of control … they're still independent contractors." (Dowling et al., 2004).

The difficulty in ensuring user choice in a primary care-led NHS is thus evident. Moreover, within the PCT the PEC wields more influence in decision-making than the Board, which it tended to think of as a rather futile body tinkering about on the margins, somewhat like an ineffectual second chamber of Parliament. While the Board struggled in some cases against this role, the alternative, should the PCT Board and PEC be at loggerheads, as they were in one instance, seemed to be for responsiveness to users to be shunted into a cul-de-sac.

Conclusion

In an early analysis of 'the Third Way' Rouse and Smith (1999) identified several key potential problems concerning its relationship with accountability. These included incoherence of the overall approach; problems of effectiveness relating to the diffusion of power; a passive citizenry; and efficiency versus democracy. These predictors have proved accurate. The tensions between central directives and local responsiveness and between a primary-care led NHS dominated by GPs and user choice and influence were present through our findings and manifested in very weak user responsiveness, neither choice in exit-terms nor voice in any meaningful way whatsoever. While going further than the Conservatives ever did in tightening managerial control on doctors, in both secondary and primary care, amounting to a return to 'Fordist' controls in some instances (Harrison and Ahmad, 2000) this has further undermined the ability of local users and citizens to exert any influence or control of their own in a local arena. The very attempt to tighten central accountability whilst devolving local decisions to users is, in policy terms, a sort of insoluble 'oxymoron' (Paton, 2006).

A return to Hirschman may shed some light on these issues and point the way to some possible path of recovery. The theory indicates that there is no defined optimal prescription for exit and/or voice; that a sort of natural decay or entropy sets in even when they have been working well, reducing voice to turn into an effectual 'blowing-off steam' and exit to become a cosy relationality. While cultural mores mean that after a certain time the effectiveness of the alternative to one dominant method may become underestimated nevertheless systems that rely upon one type of feedback may occasionally need an injection of the other, possibly in an alternating, pendulum-swing cycle.

In the new NHS, voice, the dominant mechanism for responding to users, is not working effectively. One solution for rejuvenation of user responsiveness, advocated by some (e.g. Le Grand, 2003) may be the introduction of user exit from PCTs as they once enjoyed the possibility of exiting from their GPFH. Alternatively, as others have suggested (Pickard et al., 2006) voice could be strengthened, either by placing the commissioner under professional control and making the latter accountable to patients; or by rendering PCTs representative of local communities, expressed via networks; or by mandating health commissioners to use consumer research which exists in plenty (e.g. Airey et al., 1999; Anon, 2004) to inform service agreements. As things stand, however, and hampered by the type of conflicting and contradictory accountability chains currently in place, neither of the three possibilities seem very likely. Perhaps it is New Labour itself that has to stop using 'voice' and make a choice of its own.

References

Airey, C. and Erens, B. (eds) (1999), *The National Health Services (NHS) Patients Survey*, National Centre for Social Research, London.

Anon (2004), 'Continuity of care: patients' and carers' views and choices in their use of primary care services', Unpublished research report.

Audit Commission (1996), *What the Doctor Ordered: A Study of GP Fundholders in England and Wales*, HMSO, London.

Buckland, S. and Gorin, S. (2001), *Involving Consumers? An Exploration of Consumer Involvement in NHS Research and Development Managed by Department of Health Regional Offices*, HMSO, London.

Colin-Thome, D. (1996), First Aid for Local Health Needs, *Demos*, **9**, 46–7.

Commission for Health Improvement, (CHI) (2004), *Unspeaking The Patients' Experience: Variations in the NHS Patient Experience in England*, London.

Department of Health, (2000), *The NHS Plan: A Plan for Investment,* London.

HMSO Department of Health, (2001), *Reforming the NHS Complaints Procedure: A Listening Document*, HMSO, London.

Department of Health, (2003), *Building on the Best: Choice, Responsiveness and Equity in the NHS*, HMSO, London.

Department of Health, (2004), *The NHS Improvement Plan: Putting People at the Heart of Public Services*, HMSO, London.

Dowling, B. and Glendinning, C. (2003), 'The 'new' primary care: Ideology and performance', in Dowling, B. and Glendinning, C. (2003), *The New Primary Care: Modern, Dependable, Successful?* Open University Press, Maidenhead.

Dowling, B., Sheaff, R. and Pickard, S. (2004), Governance Structures and Accountability in Primary Care, Paper presented to SIHCM conference, St, Andrew's.

Exworthy, M., Powell, M, and Mohan, J. (1999), The NHS: Quasi-Market, Quasi-hierarchy and Quasi-network? *Public Money and Management*, October–December, 15–22.

Flynn, R., Williams, G. and Pickard, S. (1996), *Markets and Networks*, Open University Press, Buckinghamshire.

Gilbert, D, (2003), 'Nothing about us without us: what patient and public involvement means to CHI', *Quality in Primary Care*, **11**, 61–5.

Harrison, A. and Dixon, J. (2000), *The NHS Facing the Future*, King's Fund, London.

Harrison, S. and Ahmad, W. (2000), Medical Autonomy and the UK State 1975 to 2025, *Sociology*, **34**(1), 129–146.

Harrison, S. and Dowswell, G. (2000), 'The selective use by NHS management of NICE-promulgated guidelines: A new and effective tool for systematic rationing of new therapies?' in Miles, A., Hampton, J. and Hurwitz, B. (eds), *NICE, CHI and the NHS Reforms: Enabling Excellence or Imposing Control?* Aesculapius Medical Press, London.

Hirschman, A.O. (1970), *Exit, Voice and Loyalty: Responses to Decline in Firms, Organizations and States*, Harvard Press, Massachusetts.

Hood, C. (1995) The 'New Public management' in the 1980s: variations on a theme, *Accounting, Organizations and Society*, **20**, 930–110

Le Grand, J. (2003), *Motivation, Agency and Public Policy*, Oxford University Press, Oxford.

Mulgan, R. (2000), '"Accountability": An ever-expanding concept?', *Public Administration*, **78**(3) 555–573.

National Health Service Executive, (NHSE) (1998), *A First Class Service: Quality in the New NHS.* Department of Health, London.

Noble, J., Hann, M., Sheaff, R. and Marshall, M. (2005), 'A survey and audit of the first "Guides to Local Health Services" produced by Primary Care Trusts in England', *Health Expectations*, **8**, 138–148.

Paton, C. (2006), *New Labour's State of Health*, Ashgate, Aldershot.

Pickard, S. and Smith, K.A. (2001), 'A Third Way for lay involvement: What evidence so far?', *Health Expectations*, **4**, 170–179.

Pickard, S., Marshall, M., Rogers, A., Sheaff, R., Sibbald, B., Campbell, S. et al., (2002), User Involvement in Clinical Governance, *Health Expectations*, **5**, 1–12.

Pickard, S., Sheaff, R. and Dowling, B. (2006), 'Exit, voice, governance and user-responsiveness', *Social Science and Medicine.*

Rhodes, RAW. (1997), *Understanding Governance*, Open University Press, Buckingham.

Robinson, B. (1996), 'Primary Managed Care: The Lyme Alternative', in Meads, G. (ed.), *Future Options for General Practice: Primary Care Development*, Radcliffe Press, Oxford.

Rouse, J. and Smith, G, (1999), 'Accountability', in Powell, M. (ed.), *New Labour, New Welfare State*, The Polity Press, Bristol.

Secretary of State for Health (2000), *The NHS Plan: A Plan for Investment, A Plan for Reform*, The Stationery Office, London.

Sheaff, R., Sibbald, B., Campbell, S., Roland, M., Marshall, M., Pickard, S., Gask, L., Rogers, A. and Halliwell, S. (2004), 'Soft governance and attitudes to clinical quality in English general practice', *Journal of Health Services Research and Policy*, **9**(3), 132–8.

Stewart, J. (1993), 'Advance of the new magistracy', Local Government Management, **1**(6), 18–19.

Young, R. and Noble, J. (2003), 'Understanding the international labour market', *Employing Doctors and Dentists*, **58**, 11–12.

Chapter 7

Fixing Legitimacy? The Case of NICE and the National Health Service

Stephen Harrison and Ruth McDonald

The National Health Service (NHS) operates on the principle that patients do not (with the exception of user charges) pay out of pocket for health care at the time of access. It thus socialises the financial risks of ill-health by pooling risk and financial provision. In theory and in practice such 'third party payment' arrangements give rise to the condition of 'consumer moral hazard' in which demand is higher than would be the case if individuals had to pay out of pocket (Donaldson and Gerard, 1993; Harrison and Hunter, 1994). Another form of moral hazard is 'supplier-induced demand'. The potential for this to occur arises from conditions in which actors proposing to supply a good or service are better able than the potential recipient to judge the latter's needs; medicine is an obvious example. Unlike consumer moral hazard, it may exist under either out of pocket or third party payment arrangements. The extent to which 'supplier-induced demand' is motivated solely by suppliers' material motives (for instance, to increase piecework earnings) is open to debate. However, it interacts with consumer moral hazard to create a situation in which neither consumer nor supplier has much incentive to moderate demand, leading to an inflation of demand (Harrison and Moran, 2000). Since resources are finite, third party payers must develop mechanisms for matching supply and demand, even in circumstances where resources are expanding. For much of its history, the NHS achieved such rationing by a combination of waiting lists, 'gatekeeping' by GPs, and the clinical autonomy of physicians, that is means largely hidden from public and patients (Harrison, 2001).

By the 1990s, this tacit arrangement was beginning to break down under several pressures. First, waiting lists were increasingly seen by government and (perhaps as a result) by the public as a mark of NHS inadequacy; the *Patient's Charter* set minimum standards and NHS institutions were penalised for failing to meet them. Second, resources were becoming tighter and in the context of managerial reforms physicians were perhaps less willing to 'play the game'. Third, the level of academic and media comment in the period 1993–96 on the topic of rationing may well have entailed a sort of 'loss of innocence'. Fourth, the logic of the quasi-market introduced in 1991 was that the purchasing bodies (Health Authorities) should prioritise expenditure from their finite budget (Harrison, 1991; McDonald, 2002). In 1993 these authorities were asked to identify interventions of which they would in future purchase more and less, on grounds of effectiveness and ineffectiveness respectively (NHS Management Executive, 1993). Some chose the insertion of grommets (a treatment for children with otitis media – 'glue ear') and dilatation and curettage ('D and C': a treatment for dysfunctional uterine bleeding) for women under the age of forty as their candidates for the 'purchase less' category (Klein et al., 1996). Both procedures had been the subject of well-publicised academic evidence reviews questioning their value (Effective Health Care, 1992, 1995). If implicit approaches seemed less tenable, the alternative was explicit rationing (McDonald, 2002). But this in turn raised further questions; who should make rationing decisions? and on what criteria should such decisions be based? A potential opportunistic answer to such questions was provided by the development in the 1990s of an 'evidence-based medicine' movement, apparently influenced by intellectual developments at McMaster University in Canada (Harrison, 1998). Although calls for NHS treatments to be more evidence-based date back at least to Cochrane's 1971 Rock Carling Lecture *Effectiveness and Efficiency: Random Reflections on Health Services* (Cochrane, 1972), the advent of the NHS Research and Development Strategy between 1991 and 1993 provided the opportunity for proponents of 'health technology assessment' to influence UK policy. By 1993 the speeches of the then Secretary of State for Health were marked by references to the R and D Programme apparently as a defence against criticisms of the quasi-market and its apparently perverse effects in such terms as non-cooperation between institutions, 'adverse selection' of patients, and the 'efficiency formula' which rewarded patient throughput without reference to quality or outcomes. These criticisms had been linked with the rationing problem described above through public and media concern at 'rationing by postcode' and more specifically by the so-called 'war of Jennifer's ear' in which capital was made in the 1992 general electoral campaign from the apparent refusal of the NHS to perform a grommet insertion for a girl with 'glue ear'.

Medical academics and politicians were thus beginning to converge on the idea that the effectiveness of medical interventions might offer a criterion for rationing that is apparently both rational and commonsensical. Yet although the Conservative government of 1992–97 did much to establish institutions to produce and review evidence of such effectiveness, such as the NHS Research and Development Programme and the Centre for Reviews and Dissemination at the University of York, it was left to the subsequent Labour government to devise an institution for implementing these principles.

The Creation and Operation of NICE

Prior to its general election victory in May 1997, the Labour Party had concentrated on criticising Conservative policies, rarely making more than the most generalised pronouncements in respect of its own policy (Labour Party, 1994, 1995). The proposal for a National Institute of Clinical Excellence (NICE) was one of several new NHS institutions announced in the white paper *The New NHS: Modern, Dependable* (Secretary of State for Health, 1997). The brief account given there focused very much on the production and dissemination of evidence-based clinical guidelines.

NICE, as envisaged at this time, was thus primarily a vehicle for influencing the practice of clinicians in line with research evidence. However, when a more detailed account of NICE's functions was published some six months later, the emphasis had changed somewhat towards national appraisal of the effectiveness and cost-effectiveness of clinical interventions and subsequent authoritative advice on what treatments should be available from the NHS (NHS Executive, 1998: 14–24). Although some emphasis was also placed on national standardisation as a means of ending 'postcode rationing', the clear intent was now for NICE to offer a nationally authoritative vehicle for rationing according to explicit criteria. It may be that this shift in emphasis was informed by the difficulties then emerging in relation to the drug Viagra, an apparently effective, but expensive treatment for male impotence (McDonald, 2000). The Secretary of State for Health, Frank Dobson, found himself in the position of pronouncing, on grounds of affordability, that only one treatment per week could be prescribed by GPs and that only for men whose condition arose from specified diseases (Klein, 2001: 214; Dodds-Smith, 2000; Dewar, 1999).

In the event, NICE was established in April 1999 with the status of a Special Health Authority and the role of undertaking 20 to 30 (originally 30 to 50) evidence-based appraisals per annum of new or existing clinical interventions. Such appraisals may result in recommendations to the Department of Health that particular treatments should not be introduced to the NHS without further trials, or in the production of 'clinical guidelines' for the management of relevant medical conditions (NHS Executive, 1998: 15–7; for more details of NICE's operation, see Syrett, 2003; Rawlins and Culyer, 2004). Appraisal is largely in the form of cost-utility analysis, that is expressed in terms of quality-adjusted life years (QALYs: for a basic account, see Edgar et al., 1998). Whilst NICE has not adopted a standard threshold for its judgements on cost-effectiveness, a retrospective analysis of appraisal determinations in its first year of operations presented at NICE's annual public meeting suggested that positive recommendations were in general associated with a cost per QALY of £30,000 or less (Raftery, 2001). Referrals to NICE take about twelve months to determine and by mid-2003, it had completed some fifty reports (www.nice.org.uk/catlist), more than thirty of which focused on pharmaceuticals and more than 10 on devices or surgical procedures. A minority (around one-fifth according a recent review – see Raftery, 2006) of appraisals have taken the form of straightforward negative recommendations, and most consist of positive endorsements, albeit with in many cases, restrictions placed on the circumstances in which the treatment should be employed. Since 2003 the NHS has been legally required to implement most NICE recommendations and the government argues that the necessary funds are included in its allocations to the Service (Shannon, 2003). A new drive to ensure compliance began in 2006 (Mayor, 2006). NICE's work has been positively evaluated in technical terms by the World Health Organisation (WHO, 2003) though more critical evaluations have been offered by the House of Commons Health Committee (2002), Maynard et al., (2004), and Devlin and Parkin (2004) and there are suggestions that the pace of NICE decision making for England is slower than that of its Scottish counterpart the Scottish Medicines Consortium, effectively reviving 'postcode rationing' (Watts, 2006).

Aside from technical and operational criteria, NICE's great challenge has been to achieve legitimacy in the eyes of public and patients, an essential requirement for such a body to retain its authority in circumstances where its decisions may effectively deny specific medical interventions to individuals who believe that they might have benefited. In fact it is clear that NICE's recommendations are not always regarded as authoritative by patients and patient groups. In part, this because much of the work of NICE's appraisals committees is conducted under terms of commercial confidentiality and may therefore be seen as lacking transparency (Kmietowicz, 2001; NICE, 2001), even in circumstances where NICE has established both wide-ranging consultation arrangements and a standing panel (the Partners Council) to represent stakeholders (Quennell, 2003). NICE has also established a Citizens Council, comprising 30 people drawn from all walks of life to help ascertain the views of members of the public on issues informing the development of NICE guidance. However, these tend to be issues of broad principle (what is need? should age-based discrimination be permissible?), rather than matters pertaining to specific appraisals. Perhaps more importantly, the widely-publicised case of Interferon Beta (a drug for relapsing-remitting Multiple Sclerosis) has shown that it is politically extremely difficult for negative recommendations to be sustained in the face of patient and pharmaceutical company demand (Syrett, 2003), having resulted in a scheme for its costs to be shared between manufacturers and the Department of Health.

A Test Case? Interferon Beta and Relapsing-remitting Multiple Sclerosis

Whilst clinical trials have shown that Interferon Beta reduces the frequency of relapse in relapsing-remitting multiple sclerosis (RRMS) patients and may influence the duration of relapse (NICE, 2002a: 4), economic evaluations of the drug suggest rather low levels of cost-effectiveness (Forbes et al., 1998; Nicholson and Milne, 1999; Parkin et al., 1998). Even before it was licensed for use in the UK, the high unit cost of the drug and estimates that it would consume ten per cent of the national drug budget (New, 1996) had begun to fuel concern at the Department of Health. Following its launch in 1996, a number of health authorities took decisions not to fund treatment, but in 1997, two months after Labour's election victory, the High Court ruled against North Derbyshire Health Authority's decision to deny it to patients (Dyer, 1997). When the work programme for NICE was produced in 1999, Interferon beta was listed as one of the first technologies to be appraised, with the NICE evaluation being a much more protracted process than initially envisaged. As NICE subsequently acknowledged 'This has been a particularly challenging appraisal, which has taken much longer than anyone involved would have wished' (NICE, 2002b).

The process began with the request from the Department of Health (DH) and the National Assembly of Wales (NAW) to appraise the drug on 6 August 1999. NICE wrote to interested parties (manufacturers, national patient/ carer groups and professional bodies) on the same day asking that any submissions to NICE regarding the drug should be made by 1 November 1999, although this deadline was subsequently extended to February 2000 following discussions between the manufacturers and DH/NAW. NICE also commissioned a review of the published evidence of clinical and cost effectiveness from the Northern and Yorkshire Drug and Therapeutic Centre. All of this information was considered at the first meeting of the Appraisal Committee held on 30 May 2000. Following this meeting the Committee then prepared its Provisional Appraisal Determination (PAD) which it circulated to consultees as strictly confidential material. However, the confidential findings of NICE's provisional appraisal of the evidence relating to Interferon beta and Glatiramer acetate, another drug for the treatment of MS, were leaked to BBC News in June 2000. The discussion of these findings in a news item on 20 June prompted NICE to issue a press release the following day confirming 'that other than for those patients who are already receiving these medicines, they should not be made available in the NHS at the present time. This is because, on the basis of a very careful consideration of the evidence, their modest clinical benefit appears to be outweighed by their very high cost.'

Meanwhile BBC News reported the comments of Peter Cardy, Chief Executive of the Multiple Sclerosis Society 'I can only say that there are going to be tens of thousands of people waking up this morning with the icy fingers of dread closing round their hearts. Sir Michael Rawlins' [Chairman of NICE] institute has taken away from them the only hope they have ever had of relief from this disease.' Shadow health secretary Liam Fox accused the government of distorting the workings of NICE by 'slipping in affordability' as one of the criteria it considered and turning NICE into an 'arms-length rationing mechanism for ministers.' In the context of emotive media images and criticism from political opponents prime minister Tony Blair responded in the House of Commons, by defending the need to consider affordability as a general principle and pointing to the large increase in NHS resources since Labour's election victory.

On 27 July the Appraisal Committee met again to consider its provisional determination in the light of feedback from consultees and agreed a Final Appraisal Determination (FAD) which was submitted to NICE. The FAD was circulated to consultees for consideration. In addition to MS patient groups, the Royal College of Nursing, the Association of British Neurologists and various pharmaceutical companies all submitted appeals against the FAD. The NICE Appeal Panel decision published in November 2000 upheld appeals in a number of areas. These included a failure on the part of the Appraisal Committee to explain the basis of its conclusion that beta interferon is 'not cost effective, when compared with alternative uses of current resources' and an acceptance that the issues relating to the long-term benefits of treatment with beta interferon may not have received full considered by the Appraisal Committee. The Appraisal Committee expressed serious reservations about the economic models submitted, but maintained that, 'on the basis of current evidence, neither beta interferon nor glatiramer is cost-effective for the NHS'. In addition, new evidence was also presented for consideration by the pharmaceutical companies manufacturing the drug. All of this resulted in a decision by NICE in December 2000 to commission further economic modelling and to extend the timeline for the evaluation process.

In January 2001 NICE wrote to consultees requesting their views on its proposals to commission the development of a new economic model and identifying where stakeholders could become involved. Manufacturers were invited to make available further data that they may have, including patient-specific data from clinical trials.

The Appraisal Committee met on 26 July 2001 to consider the results of the new economic modelling exercise and following on from this meeting produced a Provisional Appraisal Determination (PAD) which was sent to the consultees (including patient/carer organisations, professional bodies and manufacturers) on 4 August 2001. Because of speculation in the news media surrounding the content of the PAD, the Chairman on the recommendation of two of the Institute's Executive Directors, took the decision to publish the PAD on the NICE website. Further modelling took place in response to comments from consultees and the Appraisal Committee met to agree the Final Appraisal Decision on 25 October 2001 and sent this to consultees on 30 October and published it on the NICE website on 2 November 2001. Two days before this, however, the Department of Health announced that it had entered into a 'risk-sharing scheme' with the pharmaceutical companies concerned under which it would fund Interferon beta prescribing. Under this agreement the Department would fund Inteferon beta for an agreed period during which time an assessment would be made to establish the cost-effectiveness of the drug. Under this scheme, if actual benefit to patients is equal to or greater than expected benefit (a specially-increased cost per QALY threshold of £36,000), then the DH will continue to purchase the drug at the price agreed at the outset of the scheme. If however, actual benefit falls below expected, the price will be reduced to restore cost effectiveness to the expected level. (It is highly unlikely that manufacturers will be required to reimburse the government if the drug proves to be ineffective, since new drugs are likely to supersede beta interferon within a few years; Sudlow and Counsell, 2003).

NICE's response was to issue a press release immediately saying that it had had no involvement in these discussions, had no knowledge of the details and was continuing with the appraisal process. NICE published its final guidance in February 2002, setting out its reasons for recommending that beta interferon should not be funded. These focused on issues of cost-effectiveness rather than efficacy. As the guidance points out, 'In arriving at its conclusion the Appraisal Committee took account of the Directions to the Institute laid out by the Secretary of State for Health [which require NICE] to take into account inter alia the degree of clinical need of people with the condition, the broad balance of benefits and costs and the efficient use of NHS resources' (NICE, 2002a: 9).

Comments by the Liberal Democrat MP Paul Burstow MP in January 2002 suggesting that 'The fact the Department of Health is rushing out an announcement on its plans for 'risk sharing' is a vote of no confidence in NICE received a swift denial from NICE (NICE, 2002c) and by February 2002 NICE was insisting that Government had not 'over-ridden the NICE decision' since 'the [risk-sharing] scheme would not exist had not NICE undertaken its appraisal and reached the conclusion that as things stand, the drugs are not cost-effective.'(NICE, 2002b). Whilst Government has been keen to depict the risk sharing scheme as an example of evidence based medicine in action, critics suggest that the scheme is 'scientifically unsound' (Sudlow and Counsell, 2003: 388; Mayor, 2001). The planned date for reviewing the guidance on beta interferon was November 2004 on the expectation that evidence may have become available to inform a reassessment of cost-effectiveness. However, data are not expected until 2007 and although NICE has invited consultees to inform them of any evidence which might suggest that an earlier review would be beneficial

(NICE, 2004), it seems unlikely that consultees will wish to jeopardise the provision of the drug by accepting NICE's invitation. A recent report from NICE highlighted evidence that four of its guidelines, including the use of Interferon beta for multiple sclerosis had been 'over-implemented' (White, 2004).

Subsequent Developments

Subsequent developments have not suggested that NICE enjoys extensive political legitimacy. First, there has been further evidence of Government's preparedness to sidestep NICE and the rules of evidence based medicine. One example came shortly after the Interferon beta case when the Department of Health pre-empted any ruling by NICE on the drug imatinib mesylate (Glivec) for chronic myeloid leukaemia by writing to regional health directors saying that they should make funds available for the drug despite the fact that the Institute's appraisal was not expected until August 2002 (Barbour, 2001). A further example occurred in 2005 when, faced with a fierce news media debate (*Lancet*, 2005), Secretary of State for Health Patricia Hewitt instructed Primary Care Groups to fund the drug Herceptin for patients with early stage breast cancer of the HER2 positive type, despite the facts that each course of such treatment was priced at approximately £26,000, trial evidence suggested only modest benefits (Moss, 2006), and the drug had not yet been considered by NICE. Several prospective patients had also appealed to the courts (Dyer, 2006a). Accordingly, NICE undertook a fast-track appraisal, issuing favourable guidance in 2006 (Barrett et al., 2006). Second, NICE has continued to face strong opposition from patients, clinicians and drug manufacturers whenever it has attempted to reach unfavourable determinations. The major example occurred in 2006 when NICE reversed its earlier approval of drugs such as Aricept for patients in the early stages of dementia. Reaction came in the form of appeals to NICE, complaints to the Ombudsman, applications for judicial review and demonstrations by patients (Dyer, 2006b).

Perhaps none of this is surprising. As we noted above, it is well-known that third-party payment systems for health care tend to generate increases in demand, largely because they create a situation in which neither seekers (patients) nor providers (doctors and hospitals) of care have much of an incentive to moderate their demands. At some risk of hyperbole, one might say that third-party payment encourages a tacit conspiracy by patients and health care providers against third-party payers. In the UK context it is central government as third party payer, and its agents such as NICE and commissioning authorities (such as Primary Care Trusts) that have an interest in preventing the escalation of demand. Yet government cannot always simply back NICE in the face of the kind of challenges described above. In part this is because of the high political profile enjoyed by the NHS, leading to the prospect of lost votes for any party seen to damage it (Harrison and Dowswell, 2000). In part also, the government has a paradoxical relationship with the pharmaceutical industry, needing simultaneously to retain its contribution to the UK economy and to minimise NHS drugs expenditure.

It has recently been announced that NICE (renamed the National Institute for Health and Clinical Excellence, but retaining the original acronym) has been asked by the government to begin a new drive to eliminate 'ineffective and obsolete' treatments from the NHS (Foster, 2000: 6). With a few exceptions (such as the prophylactic removal of impacted wisdom teeth), NICE has to date devoted much of its effort to the appraisal of new and expensive interventions, as noted above often resulting in complex recommendations about what types of patients and stages of disease these should be used for, rather than on 'blanket bans'. It is not clear how far this new drive will take NICE into the appraisal of technologies that lead to less controversy than before. It is an unfortunate fact that interventions known to be ineffective (such as antibiotics for viral infections) continue to be demanded by patients and offered by doctors.

Perhaps in recognition of the controversy surrounding NICE guidance, NICE has published 'Social Value Judgements' (NICE, 2005) which outlines thirteen 'Principles for the Development of NICE Guidance' based on the views of the NICE Citizens' Council. Whilst some of these principles are unlikely to provoke much opposition (a refusal to discriminate on grounds of gender or sexual orientation), others are potentially very contentious (McDonald et al., 2007). For example, principle 10, which suggests that 'if self-inflicted causes ... influence the clinical or cost effectiveness of an intervention it may be appropriate to take this into account' suggests that in some cases it may be justifiable to refuse treatment to smokers if benefits of treatment are lower and/or costs higher than for non-smokers. The development of 'social value judgements' and the review of these judgements in 2007, examining issues such as the 'rule-of-rescue' and the 'problem of comborbidity', raise a number of questions: will additional groups (beyond those whose outcomes will be adversely influenced by self-inflicted causes) be singled out as appropriate for the denial of treatment? How far can the principles developed by the Citizens Council be seen as representing the views of 'ordinary' members of the public? How are these principles to be incorporated into appraisal processes which have hitherto largely focused on cost per QALY calculations? And given the contentious and protracted nature of the process to date using relatively straightforward cost-effectiveness criteria, how much more contentious, protracted and complex will the process be in the future?

References

Barbour, V. (2001), 'Imatinib for chronic myeloid leukaemia: A NICE mess', *Lancet*, **358**, 1478.

Barrett, A., Roques, T., Small, M., Smith, R.D. (2006), 'How much will Herceptin really cost?', *British Medical Journal*, **333**, 1118–20.

Cochrane, A.L. (1972), *Effectiveness and Efficiency: Random Reflections on Health Services*, Nuffield Provincial Hospitals Trust, London.

Devlin, N., Parkin, D. (2004) 'Does NICE have a cost-effectiveness threshold and what other factors influence its decisions? A binary choice model', *Health Economics*, **13**, 437–52.

Dewar, S. (1999), 'Viagra; the political management of rationing', in Appleby, J., Harrison, A. (eds), *Health care UK 1999/2000*, King's Fund, London.

Dodds-Smith, I. (2000), 'NICE and the ultimate decision makers: The legal framework for prescription and reimbursement of medicines', in Miles, A., Hampton, J.R., Hurwitz, B. (eds), *NICE, CHI and the NHS Reforms: Enabling Excellence or Imposing Control?* 103–25, Aesculapius Medical Press, London.

Donaldson, C. and Gerard, K. (1993), *The Economics of Health Care Financing: the Visible Hand*, Macmillan, London.

Dyer, C. (1997), 'Ruling on interferon beta will hit all health authorities', *British Medical Journal*, **315**, 143–148.

Dyer, C. (2006a), 'Patient is to appeal High Court ruling on breast cancer drug' *British Medical Journal*, **332**, 443.

Dyer. C. (2006b), 'NICE faces legal challenge over restriction on dementia drugs', *British Medical Journal*, **333**, 1085.

Edgar, A., Salek, S., Shickle, D. and Cohen, D. (1998), *The Ethical QALY: Ethical Issues in Health Care Resource Allocations*, Haslemere: Euromed Communications.

Effective Health Care (1992), *The Treatment of Persistent Glue Ear in Children*, University of Leeds, Leeds.

Effective Health Care (1995), *The Management of Menorrhagia*, University of Leeds Nuffield Institute for Health and University of York Centre for Reviews and Dissemination, Leeds.

Forbes, R.B., Lees, A., Waugh, N. and Swingler, R.J. (1998), 'Population-based cost-utility study of interferon-beta 1b in secondary progressive multiple sclerosis', *British Medical Journal*, **319**, 1529–33.

Foster, M. (16 September 2006), 'Weed out the waste', *BMA News*, 6.

Harrison, S. (1991), 'Working the markets: purchaser/ provider separation in English health care', *International Journal of Health Services*, **21**(4) 625–35.

Harrison, S. (1998), 'Evidence-based medicine in the NHS: Towards the history of a policy', in Skelton, R., Williamson V., *Fifty Years of the NHS: Continuities and Discontinuities in Health Policy*, University of Brighton, Brighton.

Harrison, S. (1999), 'Clinical autonomy and health policy: Past and futures', in Exworthy, M. and Halford, S. (eds), *Professionalism and the New Managerialism in the Public Sector*, Open University Press, Buckingham.

Harrison. S. (2001), 'Managing demand in the UK National Health Service', in Clark, C., McEldowney, R. (eds), *The Health Care Financial Crisis: Strategies for Overcoming an Unholy Trinity*, 31–42, Nova Science Publishers, Huntington NY.

Harrison, S., Dowswell, G. (2000), 'The selective use by NHS management of NICE-promulgated guidelines: A new and effective tool for systematic rationing of new therapies?', in Miles A., Hampton J.R., Hurwitz B. (eds), *NICE, CHI and the NHS Reforms: Enabling Excellence or Imposing Control?* 89–102, Aesculapius Medical Press, London.

Harrison S., Hunter, D.J. (1994), *Rationing Health Care*, Institute for Public Policy Research, London.

Harrison, S., Moran, M. (2000), 'Resources and rationing: managing supply and demand in health care', in Albrecht, G., Fitzpatrick, R., Scrimshaw, S. (eds), *The Handbook of Social Studies in Health and Medicine*, 493–508, Sage, New York.

House of Commons Health Committee (2002), *Health: Second Report*, http://www.publications.parliament.uk/pa/cm200102/cmselect/cmhealth/515/51502.htm.

Klein, R.E. (2001), *The New Politics of the NHS*, Pearson, Harlow.

Klein, R.E., Day, P., Redmayne, S. (1996), *Managing Scarcity: Priority Setting and Rationing in the National Health Service*, Open University Press, Buckingham.

Kmietowicz, Z. (2001), 'Reform of NICE needed to boost its credibility', *British Medical Journal*, **323**(7325) 1324.

Labour Party (1994), *Health 2000: The Health and Wealth of the Nation in the 21st Century*, London.

Labour Party (1995), *Renewing the NHS: Labour's Agenda for a Healthier Britain*, Labour Party, London.

Lancet (2005), 'Herceptin and early breast cancer: a moment for caution', *Lancet*, **366**, 1673.

Maynard, A.K., Bloor, K., and Freemantle, N. (2004), 'Challenges for the National Institute of Clinical Excellence', *British Medical Journal*, **329**, 227–9.

Mayor, S. (2001), 'Health department to fund interferon beta despite institute's ruling', *British Medical Journal*, **323**, 1087.

Mayor, S. (2006), 'Can NICE guidance be given more clout?', *British Medical Journal*, **333**, 170.

McDonald, R. (2000), 'Just say no? Drugs Politics and the UK National Health Service', *Policy and Politics*, **28**(4) 563–576.

McDonald, R. (2002), *Using Health Economics in Health Services: Rationing Rationally?* Open University Press, Buckingham.

McDonald, R., Mead, N., Cheraghi-Sohi, S. Bower, P. and Whalley, D. (2007) Governing the ethical consumer: identity, choice and the primary care medical encounter, *Sociology of Health and Illness*, **29**(4) 1–27.

Moss, S. (4 March 2006), Hype and Herceptin, *New Scientist*, http://www.martinfrost.ws/htmlfiles/wonder_drugs2.html.

National Institute for Clinical Excellence (2001), Press Release, 2001/040 NICE Response to Consumers' Association Briefing Paper, http://www.nice.org.uk/page.aspx?o=25329.

National Institute for Clinical Excellence (2002a), Multiple sclerosis: Beta interferon and glatiramer acetate: Technology Appraisal Guidance, http://www.nice.org.uk/pdf/Multiple%20Sclerosis%20Final%20Guidance.pdf.

National Institute for Clinical Excellence (2002b), Some common questions, and their answers, resulting from the NICE guidance on the use of beta interferon and glatiramer acetate for multiple sclerosis, http://www.nice.org.uk/page.aspx?o=27641.

National Institute for Clinical Excellence (2002c), Press Release. 2002/004 NICE responds to comments made by Mr Paul Burstow MP, http://www.nice.org.uk/page.aspx?o=26969.

National Institute for Clinical Excellence (2004), Multiple sclerosis: beta interferon and glatiramer acetate (No. 32), Review proposal, http://www.nice.org.uk/pdf/MS_review_1204.pdf.

National Institute for Health and Clinical Excellence (2005), Social Value Judgments, http://www.nice.org.uk/page.aspx?o=283494.

New, B. (1996), 'The Rationing Agenda in the NHS', *British Medical Journal*, **312**, 1593–1601.

NHS Executive (1998), *A First Class Service: Quality in the New NHS*, Department of Health, London.

NHS Management Executive (1993), *Purchasing for Health: A Framework for Action*, Leeds NHS Management Executive Unit.

Nicolson, T., Milne, R. (1999), *Beta interferons (1a and 1b) in relapsing-remitting and secondary progressive multiple sclerosis*, Development and Evaluation Committee Report No 98, Wessex Institute for Health Research and Development, Southampton.

Parkin, D.W., McNamee, P., Jacoby, A., Miller, P., Thomas, S. and Bates, D. (1998), A cost-utility analysis of interferon beta for multiple sclerosis, *Health Technology Assessment*, **2**(4).

Quennell P. (2003), 'Getting a word in edgeways? Patient group participation in the appraisal process of the National Institute for clinical Excellence', *Clinical Governance International*, **8**(2) 39–45.

Raftery, J. (2001), 'NICE: faster access to modern treatments? Analysis of guidance on health technologies', *British Medical Journal*, **323**, 1300–3.

Raftery, J. (2006). 'Review of NICE's recommendations, 1999–2005', *British Medical Journal*, **332**, 1266–1268.

Rawlins, M.D., Culyer, A.J. (2004), 'National Institute for Clinical Excellence and its value judgements', *British Medical Journal*, **329**, 224–7.

Secretary of State for Health (1997), *The New NHS: Modern, Dependable*, Cm. 3807, The Stationery Office, London.

Shannon, C. (2003), NICE annual conference, *British Medical Journal*, **327**, 1368.

Sudlow, C., Counsell, C. (2003), 'Problems with UK Government's Risk Sharing Scheme for Assessing Drugs for Multiple Sclerosis', *British Medical Journal*, **326**, 388–392.

Syrett, K. (2003), 'A technocratic fix to the "legitimacy" problem? The Blair government and health care rationing in the United Kingdom', *Journal of Health Politics, Policy and Law*, **28**(4) 715–46.

Watts, G. (2006), 'Are the Scots getting a better deal on prescribed dugs than the English?', *British Medical Journal*, **333**, 875.

White, C. (2004), 'NICE guidance has failed to end "postcode prescribing"', *British Medical Journal*, **328**, 1277.

Chapter 8

Nothing New under the Sun? Regimes of Public Representation in the English National Health Service: Past, Present and Future

Anna Coleman and Stephen Harrison

Until the reorganisation of the English National Health Service in 1974, the various institutions that administered it were also responsible for representing the public. Even though directly elected local government authorities provided only the public health and community services elements of the NHS, the appointed hospital management committees and executive councils for the family health services (general medical, dental and optical practitioners and pharmacists) had been assumed to be responsible both for managing the service and for representing the user and public interest. Indeed, some members of such authorities had chosen to take, though apparently rather ineffectively, a service user viewpoint (Levitt and Wall, 1984: 254). However, the area and regional health authorities created to run the newly-unified service from 1974 onwards were responsible only for its management (Levitt and Wall, 1984: 254), an arrangement that has survived the numerous subsequent reorganisations of these institutions. Since that time, the public representation function has been carried out by separate bodies, Community Health Councils (CHCs) from 1974 until their abolition in 2003, and since then by local government authorities exercising their responsibility for 'overview and scrutiny' of the NHS (hereafter 'health scrutiny').

In this chapter, we compare these two regimes of representation in terms of their operation, origins and impact. Neither regime has been extensively studied by empirical researchers, so that for CHCs we draw on a small number of published studies and for health scrutiny on our own recent work (Coleman and Harrison, 2006). Our focus here is upon ongoing and general arrangements for public involvement in the NHS. We do not therefore consider regimes of *patient* involvement, whose logic and stakes differ from those of the public (Harrison et al., 2002) nor the more *ad hoc* approaches to public consultation such as the National Institute for Clinical Excellence's 'citizens' council' (Davies et al., 2005) or the 'citizens' juries' (e.g. Barnes 1999), and 'health panels' (e.g. Mort et al., 1999) employed in some localities. The structure of the chapter is as follows. The first two sections respectively describe and review evidence about CHCs and health scrutiny, and a third section examines the inferences that may be drawn from this comparison. A fourth section summarises the recent flurry of policy activity in the field of public involvement, whilst brief concluding remarks assess their implications.

Community Health Councils

CHCs were invented to fill a political vacuum. As noted above, the health authorities created under the 1974 NHS reorganisation were appointed with specific management responsibilities, in the then prevailing belief that there would otherwise be a dangerous confusion of roles as had contributed, for instance, to the 1969 scandal over mistreatment of patients at Ely Hospital (Klein and Lewis, 1976: 14–15). Moreover, the new authorities were smaller than their predecessors, with less scope for lay participation. However, it became necessary, expectations of local community involvement having been aroused, to provide a mechanism for the restoration of local participation (Webster, 1996: 460), so that CHCs came to be

> invented almost by accident because, when the plans for a reorganised [NHS] were almost complete, all those involved realised that something was missing: an element which could be ... seen as providing a degree of local democracy, consumer participation or public involvement (Klein and Lewis, 1976: 11).

Klein and Lewis go on to note that CHCs' subsequent evolution and uncertainties about their role reflected this improvised beginning.

The CHCs, one for each NHS district, had the role of representing the views of local public and patients to the relevant health authorities. Half of the membership was nominated by local government authorities, one-third by voluntary organisations, and the remaining one-sixth by regional health authorities. The CHCs also had powers to co-opt additional members (Levitt and Wall, 1984: 254–55) and select their own chairpersons (Hallas, 1976: 13). The early members of CHCs were not sociologically or demographically representative of the population; the middle-aged, the middle class and males were over-represented in total, though not to the same extent in every region (Klein and Lewis, 1976: 29–36). Throughout their life, CHCs were criticised as being dominated by white, middle class, middle aged people, out of touch with and unknown to the local community (Cooper et al., 1995; Baggott, 2005).

Between 1974 and 2003 CHCs were the official bodies representing the interests in the NHS of their local public (Levitt, 1980: 10), and to make representations and recommendations for improvements to the authorities responsible for managing the services. CHCs were expected to cover all aspects of the NHS and had the following rights:

- To be consulted by the local health authority on substantial changes to the patterns of health care in the district;
- To enter and inspect the premises of NHS providers;
- To receive from the NHS such information as is necessary to carry out their duties; and
- To refer to the Secretary of State for Health any proposals with which they disagreed.

CHCs were not responsible for the investigation of individual patient complaints, but could give advice to patients as to how pursue them (Levitt, 1980: 18).

Though the existence and role of CHCs remained controversial in some quarters, they narrowly escaped abolition in 1982 (Webster, 1998: 143, 160) and the 1991 reorganisation of the NHS, which introduced the so-called 'internal market' (Harrison, 1991), retained them in unchanged form, but with their role broadened from voicing the views of the community to include closer working with purchasers (health authorities and GP fundholders) to identify local needs, monitor and develop services, help to develop and monitor the *Patient's Charter*, help hospitals to obtain patients' views and monitor patterns of complaints. However, they received no extra funds to perform this expanded role (Cooper et al., 1995) and indeed their powers were subsequently defined more narrowly than before (Levitt and Wall, 1992: 288). In addition, the development of new regimes of performance management and other methods of involving the public contributed to their marginalisation (Pickard, 1997).

There was considerable diversity between CHCs both in specific work that they undertook and in their general approach (Hallas, 1976; Day and Klein, 1985; Cooper et al., 1995), but such studies as exist suggest that, despite some successes (Levitt, 1980; Webster, 1996: 634), CHCs did not have a significant overall impact (Hallas, 1976: 59; Klein and Lewis, 1976: 135; Levitt, 1980; Schulz and Harrison, 1983: 30–33; Lee and Mills, 1982: 142; Williamson, 1992: 78; Lupton et al., 1995; Cooper et al., 1995; Pickard, 1997; Baggott, 2005). They were poorly resourced, sometimes overwhelmed with work, often torn between how much effort to devote to influencing NHS plans and how much to respond to dissatisfactions expressed by individuals. Few felt able to enquire into the standards of clinical care offered by local providers. CHC members differed as to how far their role was to represent the community to NHS managers and how far to form a diplomatic bridge between the two. They were often thought unimportant by NHS managers, who felt that they themselves already had better information about local health care needs and conducted consultation exercises that left CHCs with impossibly short deadlines. CHCs that were deemed to have forfeited NHS management goodwill were subsequently by-passed in consultations, whilst those deemed to have been more co-operative were used by health authorities as part of their own 'legitimation strategy'. Some health authorities tried to persuade (unwilling) CHCs to undertake consultations about health care rationing priorities. The legitimacy of CHCs may also have been undermined by the attendance difficulties of their local government authority members, and the difficulties they experienced in involving either the public or the wider field of voluntary organisations. Finally, the ability of CHCs to influence service changes (such as forcing referral to the Secretary of State) was largely confined to hospital care, and was in any case progressively attenuated by various changes in national regulations and by local managerial strategies such as declaring emergency bed closures.

In summary, CHCs were dogged by problems of legitimacy, resources and powers (Baggott, 2005) whilst addressing an expanding agenda (Lupton, et al., 1995) and without clear guidelines for operation or agreed criteria for assessing effectiveness (Ham, 1986; Hogg, 1993). English CHCs (though not their Welsh equivalents) were abolished by the Labour government in December 2003 (Department of Health, 2003).

Health Overview and Scrutiny

Local authority health scrutiny came about as a direct, initially unintended result of the replacement in most local government authorities of the traditional system in which much decision making took place in functional executive committees in which all elected councillors participated (Stoker et al., 2003). The new system, introduced by the Local Government Act of 2000, provided for decision-making by a much smaller group (sometimes referred to as a 'cabinet') of 'executive' councillors, leaving the need to define a role for 'non-executive' councillors. The notion of 'overview and scrutiny committees' (OSCs) consequently emerged; on which non-executive councillors were to act effectively as 'backbenchers' scrutinising decisions and council services and holding the Executive to account. The Local Government Act 2000 also introduced the concept of 'community leadership', giving local authorities a new duty to promote the economic, social and environmental well-being of local communities. Commensurate with this new role, OSCs were also able to scrutinise the work of external service providers that might impact on the well-being of the local population. The Social Care Act of 2001 gave OSCs in top-tier local authorities the power to scrutinise the NHS. It is important to note that the legislation was far from prescriptive about the precise arrangements to be adopted. Thus all social services local authorities must have an OSC, composed of elected non-executive councillors, that can respond to proposals to change services from the NHS, but it is left for each authority to decide whether and how to bundle health scrutiny in its wider allocation of scrutiny responsibilities to its various OSCs. Moreover, the non-executive role is new and challenging for councillors used to participation in the executive committees of the previous local government regime (Centre for Public Scrutiny, 2002). OSCs have the discretion to set their own agendas for undertaking detailed scrutiny of health issues (including the NHS) if they so choose and can call representatives of NHS bodies to give evidence to them.

According to the Centre for Public Scrutiny 'effective patient and public involvement needs to be carried out across three levels:

- the individual – involving patients or carers in decisions about their own care and treatment, or that of another person;
- the collective – involving patients, carers and the public in decisions about planning and delivery of services;
- the strategic – involving patients, carers and the public in longer term, strategic issues, rather than service issues' (2005: 5).

OSCs operate mainly at the collective and strategic levels. They focus on creating improvement across health services and look at the experience of individuals where they can be seen to reflect the experience of groups. OSCs do not become involved in individual complaints about treatment or care (which are the responsibility of the

Patient Advice and Liaison Services in each Primary Care and NHS Trust and the Independent Complaints Advocacy Service), though they may consider scrutinising how trends in complaints influence service improvement. There is, however, some potential overlap between the role of OSCs and those of the Patient and Public Involvement Forums (PPIFs) currently organised within each Trust. However, it is with OSCs that the NHS must undertake statutory consultations about major service developments and variations. Given the newness of health scrutiny as an institution and the relative novelty of the roles of participants, it is perhaps not surprising that quite diverse approaches have been adopted. Our research (Coleman and Harrison, 2006) suggests that, although health scrutiny structures have been successfully established, the process has generally suffered from a lack of resourcing (training, officer support and recognition of the process by council executives, NHS bodies and the public), the non-prescriptive nature of guidance for scrutiny, and confusion about the respective roles of OSCs and other institutions of public and patient involvement mentioned above. Participants also perceived an ambiguity in key definitions, especially concerning what are to be regarded as substantial developments and variations to services. Of course, OSCs are subject to membership instability resulting from (usually annual) local government elections. Difficulties have also been caused by the sheer volume of statutory consultations from the NHS, and we found little evidence of systematic direct involvement of patients or the public in the health scrutiny process. Many health OSCs initially struggled to link effectively to other involvement structures at a local level, though by 2005 they were beginning to build links with PPIFs. Nevertheless, review topics have developed over the last three or four years to include broader, cross-cutting, health improvement issues as well as specific organisations and services. A particularly important finding has been that the various parties involved in health scrutiny have, except in the case of statutory consultations, predominantly chosen to use the process integratively as an opportunity to build inter-agency networks and co-operative relationships rather than adversarially as the means of invigorating democratic debate and challenge (Coleman 2006). Some 'process benefits', such as new partnerships, the consolidation of evidence about particular review topics and more structured consideration of statutory consultation topics have flowed from health scrutiny (Bradshaw et al., 2005, Smith et al., 2006), but the choice of this approach makes it particularly difficult to assess the impact of health scrutiny in terms of changes to services or organisation that would otherwise have not occurred.

Past and Present

Though both ostensibly designed to fulfil the same broad purpose, that is to offer a vehicle for popular influence on the NHS, partly through connecting to local government, CHCs and OSCs are very different institutions. For most of their existence, CHCs had a virtual monopoly of their function, whilst OSCs exist in crowded and rapidly-changing representational environment. CHCs were constitutionally linked to the voluntary sector, whilst the membership of OSCs is a monopoly of elected local politicians. CHCs were very much NHS-centred, whilst

OSCs have been able to pursue a wider brief. Moreover, the organisational contexts of CHCs and OSCs differ; it is likely that OSCs have a degree of legitimacy for NHS managers who work in a much less insular environment than the NHS of the 1970s. Yet the 'careers' of CHCs and of OSCs to date do exhibit some parallels. First, both institutions seem to have been conceived as afterthoughts, the consequences of other, more carefully planned reorganisations undertaken for clearer purposes. Second, and perhaps partly as a consequence, both institutions have exhibited uneven patterns of development and substantial local variation. Third, neither institution found it easy to build links with their local publics. Fourth, neither institution has evidently exerted substantial influence on the content, pattern or organisation of health services (though we might concede that it is perhaps too early to rule out future possibilities for greater OSC impact). Fifth, both institutions faced strategic choices about how far to present an adversarial stance towards NHS management, either strategy presenting undesired consequences: respectively branding as 'troublemakers', or co-optation into management agendas and purposes. Whilst these poles have usually been avoided, the impression given by the evidence is that the choices made have generally been towards the latter.

What are we to make of this comparison? We might most of all infer a high level of puzzlement on the part of the designers of policy over the years. First, whilst no doubt every policy maker would aspire to involvement policies serving to legitimise the NHS as an institution and the role of government in maintaining it, it is less clear whether they have wished to develop arrangements that seriously challenge managerial or professional dominance, especially where public opinion runs counter to central priorities. (The previous chapter by Harrison and McDonald in this volume illustrates this dilemma perfectly.) Second, it is hardly clear whether policy makers have wanted the numerous institutions of health and social care to co-operate or to challenge each other. There is a good deal of evidence, from studies of CHCs and of health scrutiny and of the NHS more generally (see, for instance, Flynn et al., 1996), that the institutions have generally chosen co-operation. Third, the invention of involvement arrangements, as it were 'on the hoof', suggests a lack of confidence as to how to create the desired situation. We shall see in the next section that this process of invention has increased in speed. Finally, there is ample evidence of puzzlement at local level too. Numerous studies of 'involvement' in addition to those cited above have shown relatively little success in engaging the public on an ongoing and systematic basis (see, for instance, Milewa et al., 2002).

Further Developments

Policy related to public involvement in health shows no sign of stabilising. During 2006 three major policy documents were published which will potentially have far reaching impacts on local authority scrutiny of health.

First, Chapter 7 of the health white paper *Our Health, Our Care, Our Say* (Secretary of State for Health, 2006) discusses issues of accountability, influence and public involvement. The White Paper aspires to create health and social care services which are, regardless of who provides them, user centered, responsive, flexible, open to challenge, accountable to communities and constantly open to improvement, suggesting that this might be achieved by:

- Placing a duty on commissioners and providers 'systematically and rigorously' to discover what people want, especially difficult to reach groups;
- Establishing a Patient and Public Involvement Resource Centre;
- Expecting elected local councilors to act as advocates for their local communities ('Community call for action').
- 'Local triggers' relating to public satisfaction and service quality will require Primary Care Trusts to take action where it is evident that local needs are not being met. Evidence will be drawn from inspections, assessments by Strategic Health Authorities and by using inequality indicators.

Second, the consultation document A *Stronger Local Voice* (Department of Health, 2006) sets out plans to abolish PPIFs and in their place establish Local Involvement Networks (LINks) for every social service local authority area. These arrangements will therefore be area based rather than organisation based, and will be funded through local authorities. It is proposed that LINks will 'establish special relationships' with OSCs and will have the power to refer matters to the OSC and expect an appropriate response. The co-terminosity of LINks with local authority boundaries may help facilitate relationships with health OSCs. It is also proposed that Health OSCs will be encouraged to focus their attention on service commissioners, rather than providers. This will be especially important in terms of the developing practice-based commissioning processes. Commissioners will have a duty to respond to the community (the local triggers described above) in addition to the existing requirements to consult and involve them in changes to services locally. LINks will have statutory powers to require both NHS and social care bodies to provide requested information and respond to recommendations and are currently being piloted in selected early adopter areas.

Third, the local government white paper *Strong and Prosperous Communities* (Secretary of State for Communities and Local Government, 2006), aspires to strengthen local leadership, enhance the role of local councillors, cut back on national targets, streamline inspection, broaden the scope of Local Area Agreements and give local people greater influence in order to improve their lives. It contains proposals to strengthen overview and scrutiny, including:

- extending the remit of scrutiny to other service providers;
- extending the Community Call for Action to all local government matters;
- encouraging more use of 'area' based OSCs;
- extending the use of co-option onto OSCs; and
- encouraging councils to dedicate resources to support scrutiny.

Many public service providers, including PCTs, police and fire authorities, probation boards, passenger transport authorities and regional development agencies, will be covered by a duty to co-operate. This includes the requirement to appear before an OSC or provide specified information (in relation to service delivery) within 20 days of a request (corresponding to the Freedom of Information Act) and a right for OSCs to recommend an independent inspection of services where it is seen as necessary. Health OSCs will additionally be encouraged to scrutinise the responses of local authorities and PCTs to annual reports of the Directors of Public Health. OSCs will be encouraged to promote co-option onto committees to widen knowledge and spread the burden of any additional work and proposals for reducing or abolishing Best Value reviews may free up OSC time.

Concluding Remarks

The new arrangements for public involvement, whilst apparently continuing to invent institutions 'on the hoof', contain an important consistent philosophy insofar as they seem to address 'cross-cutting' issues by virtue of being geographically, rather than organisationally based. At the same time, they seem to emphasise challenge as much as co-operation, so that it remains to be seen whether a focus on cross-cutting, inter-agency issues can easily be maintained in such an environment. The new arrangements also apparently seek to focus (in the terms of the Centre for Public Scrutiny quoted above) on 'strategic' planning issues rather than on services more concretely. This is most evident in the proposed focus on commissioning rather than on provision, and raises two questions. First, how far will this new focus assist the already puzzling task of involving the public? If it is already difficult to recruit the public to the discussion of concrete facilities and specific services, how much more difficult will it be to raise an ongoing interest in strategic abstractions? Second, how far will the fact that the main focus of public involvement will now be on the 'middlemen' (commissioners) rather than on service providers strengthen or weaken its influence? The answer is not self-evident, but there is at least a danger that the organisational distancing of providers from public will weaken the influence (such as it is) of the latter. The puzzles that have characterised this area of health policy remain.

References

Baggott, R. (2005), 'A funny thing happened on the way to the forum? Reforming patient and public involvement in the NHS in England', *Public Administration*, **83**(3) 533–51.

Barnes, M. (1999), *Building a Deliberative Democracy: An Evaluation of Two Citizens' Juries*, Institute for Public Policy Research, London.

Bradshaw, D., Coleman, A., Gains, F., Smith, L., Greasley, S. and Boyd, A. (2005), *Process, Progress and Making it Work: Health Overview and Scrutiny in England*, Executive Summary, Centre for Public Scrutiny, London.

Centre for Public Scrutiny (2002), *Better scrutiny for better government*, downloaded from: www.idea.gov.uk/scrutiny.

Centre for Public Scrutiny (2005), *Local Authority Health Overview and Scrutiny Committees and Patient and Public Involvement Forums: A Practical Guide*, Centre for Public Scrutiny, London.

Coleman, A.J. (2006), 'Health scrutiny, democracy and integration: part of the same jigsaw?' *Local Government Studies*, **32**(2) 123–38.

Coleman, A.J. and Harrison, S. (2006), *The Implementation of Local Authority Scrutiny of Primary Health Care: 2002–2005*, University of Manchester National Primary Care Research and Development Centre, Manchester.

Cooper, E., Coote, A., Davies, A. and Jackson, C. (1995), *Voices Off: Tackling the Democratic Deficit in Health*, Institute for Public Policy Research, London.

Davies, C., Wetherell, M., Barnett, E. and Seymour-Smith, S. (2005), *Opening the Box: Evaluating the Citizens Council of NICE*, Open University School of Health and Social Welfare, Milton Keynes.

Day, P., Klein, R.E. (1985), Central accountability and local decision making: Towards the new NHS, *British Medical Journal*, **290**, 1676–8.

Department of Health (2003), Abolition of Community Health Councils: ministerial statement, downloaded from: http://www.doh.gov.uk/involvingpatients/ministerialstatement.htm.

Department of Health (2006), *A Stronger Local Voice: A Framework for Creating A Stronger Local Voice in the Development of Health and Social Care Services*, Department of Health, London.

Flynn, R., Williams, G. and Pickard, S. (1996), *Markets and Networks: Contracting in Community Health Services*, Open University Press, Buckingham.

Hallas, J. (1976), *CHCs in Action*, Nuffield Provincial Hospitals Trust, London.

Ham, C.J. (1986), *Handbook for Community Health Council Members*, University of Bristol School for Advanced Urban Studies, Bristol.

Harrison, S. (1991), Working the markets: purchaser/provider separation in English health care, *International Journal of Health Services*, **21**(4) 625–35.

Harrison, S., Milewa, T. and Dowswell, G. (2002), 'Public and user "involvement" in the National Health Service', *Health and Social Care in the Community*, **10**(2) 63–6.

Hogg, C. (1993), *Performance Standards for CHCs: Developing a Framework*, ACHCEW, London.

Klein, R.E. and Lewis, J. (1976), *The Politics of Consumer Representation*, Centre for Studies in Social Policy, London.

Lee, K., Mills, A. (1982), *Policy-Making and Planning in the Health Sector*, Croom Helm, London.

Levitt, R. (1980), *The People's Voice in the NHS*, King Edward's Hospital Fund for London, London.

Levitt, R. and Wall, A. (1984), *The Reorganised National Health Service*, (3rd edn), Croom Helm, London.

Levitt, R. and Wall, A. (1992), *The Reorganised National Health Service*, (4th edn), Chapman and Hall, London.

Lupton, C., Buckland, S. and Moon, G. (1995), 'Consumer involvement in health care purchasing: The role and influence of Community Health Councils', *Health and Social Care in the Community*, **3**(4) 215–26.

Milewa, T., Harrison, S., Ahmad, W.I.U. and Tovey, P. (2002), '"Citizens" participation in primary health care planning: Innovative citizenship practice in empirical perspective', *Critical Public Health*, **12**(1) 39–53.

Mort, M., Harrison, S., Dowswell, T. (1999), 'Public Health Panels: Influence at the Margin', in Khan, U.A. (ed.), *Participation Beyond the Ballot Box: European Case Studies in State-Citizen Political Dialogue*, 94–109, UCL Press, London.

Pickard, S. (1997), 'The future organisation of Community Health Councils', *Social Policy and Administration*, **32**, 226–44.

Schulz, R.I. and Harrison, S. (1983), *Teams and Top Managers in the National Health Service*, King's Fund, London.

Secretary of State for Communities and Local Government (2006), *Strong and Prosperous Communities*, Cm 6939, The Stationery Office, London.

Secretary of State for Health (2006), *Our Health, Our Care, Our Say: A New Direction for Community Health Services*, Cm 6737, The Stationery Office, London.

Smith, E., Shacklady-Smith, A. and Bradshaw, D. (2006), *Sharing the Learning: Lessons from Health Scrutiny in Action*, Centre for Public Scrutiny, London.

Stoker, G., Gains, F., John, P., Rao, N. and Harding, A. (2003), *Implementing the 2000 Act with Respect to New Council Constitutions and the Ethical Framework: First Report*, London: Office of the Deputy Prime Minister (http://www.elgce.org.uk).

Webster, C. (1996), *The Health Services Since the War: Volume II – Government and Health Care: The British National Health Service 1958–1979*, HMSO, London.

Webster, C. (1998), *The National Health Service: A Political History*, Oxford University Press, Oxford.

Williamson, C. (1992), *Whose Standards? Consumer and Professional Standards in Health Care*, Open University Press, Buckingham.

Chapter 9

Two Cheers for Public Health

Chris Nottingham

Since 1997 Scottish Executive health pronouncements have reflected values and approaches associated with the New Public Health (NPH). *Our National Health* (*Scottish Executive*, 2000) warned 'better health cannot be achieved just by Government regulation or by spending more money ... We must change the culture of health and healthcare services to give people better healthcare services and make Scotland a healthier nation.' This required 'national effort' (*Scottish Executive*, 2000: 3): 'Health is not just Government's responsibility. It is everyone's responsibility. As a nation, we cannot simply legislate or spend our way to better health' (*Scottish Executive*, 2000: 11). A change of direction was indicated: 'For too long, health policy and health services have focused on the treatment of ill health rather than on its prevention', and, as if to underline its NPH credentials, the paper repeated the core mantra, 'we are committed to making the NHS a national *health* service, not a national illness service' (*Scottish Executive*, 2000: 18). Professionals in the new model are enlisted as promoters of health. Individuals consulting health care professionals can expect something more than treatments for complaint they went in with. After a recent development, even a toothache could involve wider issues, as dentists have been enlisted to look for the tell tale signs of heavy alcohol consumption in their patients' mouths and refer them to their GPs (*Sunday Times* Scotland, 14 January 2007).

Partnership for Care. Scotland's White Paper hammered home the same points, linking them with 'a step change in health improvement' (*Scottish Executive*, 2003: 7). The new managed clinical networks were presented as active instruments designed for these ends. Patients were encouraged to think of themselves 'as partners in their own health care' (*Scottish Executive*, 2003: 8). NHS Scotland would be dedicated to 'Supporting and empowering patients', though professionals were apparently to be empowered at the same time. 'Staff are the health service and it is only through empowering and supporting them that services can be improved in ways that patients need' (*Scottish Executive*, 2003: 8). Staff, however will not be sufficiently empowered to escape 'tightened national guidelines', although the Paper insisted, 'we explicitly reject a command and control management approach' (*Scottish Executive*, 2003: 9). National efforts were to be extended beyond the conventional sites. Help was offered for 'small and medium sized enterprises in dealing with drug and alcohol problems among employees.'(*Scottish Executive*, 2003: 14). Balancing the promise to take 'the Patient's point of view' there was mention of 'patient's responsibilities' and a statement that 'Genuine partnership will depend on changes in cultures and behaviours on both sides', but the implications were not developed. (*Scottish Executive*, 2003:

21) *Reducing Health Inequalities: An Action Report* involved a similar ambiguity. It promised 'a whole systems approach' while insisting that the business would be 'person centred'. It is all too easy to score logical points against politicians and those who write on their behalf. Political responsibility denies its holders the privilege of frank expression and ambiguity can serve decent ends. However the evangelical tone that discourages dissent and transcends potential conflicts must be noted.

Another indication of the Executive's commitment to public health approaches was the appointment of Harry Burns, the former Director of Public Health for Greater Glasgow and a campaigner on health equality issues, as Chief Medical Officer. His first report (NHS Scotland, 2006) contained few references to health care. It led with breast feeding, road safety instruction, immunisation, and the ban on smoking in public places. Burns also promised to 're-energise efforts to convince Scots of the significant harm to health caused by excessive consumption of alcohol' (NHS Scotland, 2006: 1) the issue around which the NPH lobby is currently rallying. A very public indication of the enthusiasm for the new approach was the way the smoking ban in public places was embraced by the First Minister. McConnell has been unequivocal in his support and anxious to present the policy as a key indicator of how a devolved administration can produce solutions tailored to Scottish needs.

It would be wrong to suggest that the embrace of NPH approaches was unique to Scotland but its rise has been more rapid and less equivocal in Edinburgh than in London. There are a number of reasons for this. First, Scotland's poor comparative position in health outcomes, a fixed centre of Scottish health discourses for many years, make such statements as, 'It is time to stop making Scotland a case study in ill health and instead make it a showcase for good health'(*Scottish Executive*, 2000: 10) is difficult to oppose. Secondly, an interventionist approach to population health suggests demonstrable benefit arising from the devolution arrangements. In this context a vigorous pursuit of population health is attractive. As *Our National Health* put it 'The creation of the Scottish Parliament and the development of this Plan are inextricably linked. They have "grown up" together' (*Scottish Executive*, 2000: 9). Thirdly, the appeal of such policies owes something to the special place which health holds in the new Scottish politics. 'Since the Scottish Parliament was established, health and NHS issues have been to the fore more than any other policy area' (*Scottish Executive*, 2000: 9). Health is by far the most important responsibility of the *Scottish Executive* in terms of both costs (broadly defined the health budget accounts for more than a third of total expenditure) and the intensity of public interest in the issue. Unfortunately, the delivery of health care is a zone of perpetual difficulty. The Scottish media, like the English, present a steady flow of stories about poor service, 'super bug' infections, hospital and unit closures and the puzzling failure of greatly increased spending to produce visible improvement. In the face of the battle to match population needs and rising expectations with escalating costs, public health initiatives promise some respite. The smoking ban for instance offered an opportunity to demonstrate vigorous action in pursuit of a relatively popular end at minimal cost. Broader potential costs, and the tasks of enforcement were substantially transferred onto others. Flooding the media with injunctions to individuals to consume five units of fruit or vegetables a day, may or may not produce the desired end, but compared with the task of delivering acceptable healthcare it is a low cost means of creating an impression of purposeful action.

However while current domestic factors and different traditions (Stewart, 2004) may help explain why Scotland assimilated NPH rhetoric so readily there are underlying factors that make the shift an appealing option for policy makers in many regimes and policies need to be understood in the broader context.

Decline, Fall and Rise

Thus recent prominence of public health in the UK is often presented as a rise from the ashes. The most familiar story suggests that with the foundation of the NHS public health perspectives suffered a serious decline. Medical Officers of Health suffered declining status and such areas as occupational health were neglected. Attention and expectation became focused on the doctor-led health care sector, boosted by new drug technologies and dominated by a glamorous hospital sector, while public health professionals languished in the drab municipal sector. Recent contributions suggest that the depths were not reached until the 1970s. For Ashton, a key figure in the development of NPH, it was the NHS reorganisation of 1974 that brought 'loss of capacity and the loss of coherence' in public health. The local authority public health departments lacked glamour but retained capacity. Liverpool for example in the 1950s had over 5000 such staff. 'We are talking about health visitors, nurses, social workers, environmental health, food hygiene and so on. It was huge' (Berridge, 2006: 50). But the 1974 reorganisation brought fragmentation and reduced the effectuality of these professions. For Ashton, as Medical Officer, his power base, 'in the sense of bodies on the street', was gone. A former chair of the Hampshire Area Health Authority regarded 1974 as a 'disaster' for public health (Berridge, 2006: 18). The Labour Government in 1976 did issue the consultative document *Prevention and Health: Everybody's Business* that discussed health inequalities, road accidents, smoking, alcohol, and mental health, but, the subsequent white paper was a 'cautious' document (Cmd. 7047, 1977; Baggott, 2000: 51).

At this point it is useful to consider definitions. In reality public health is far greater than the concept discussed here. A check of public health journals quickly reveals that the controversial parts of the discipline are no more than the tip of the tip of an iceberg. Ann Tacket perceptively summarised the activities of NPH advocates as 'public health round the edges' (Berridge, 2006: 16). Public health in the menu of definitions assembled by Baggott (Baggott, 2000: 1–2) can include the 'science and art of preventing disease', promoting health and efficiency through sanitation, clean water, and education, the 'organisations of medical and nursing services for early diagnosis and preventive treatment of disease' as well as 'the development of social machinery which will ensure to every individual in the community a standard of living adequate for the maintenance of health'. As Baggott commented, 'a very broad church indeed' (Baggott, 2000: 1). Proponents of NPH do not separate themselves from the longer tradition of immunisation, food inspection, and public health medicine. Indeed they recognise the periodic safety crises such as the disastrous salmonella outbreak at Stanley Royd hospital in 1984 or e coli outbreak at a Wishaw butcher's shop (Berridge, 2006: 52–3) as an opportunity to advance the cause, but their enthusiasm, as befits practical idealists, is focused on the growth points derived from their core agenda; the promotion of a 'social model' of health and a critique of the limitations of the 'medical model', the adoption of targets for population health based on international epidemiological comparisons, the reduction of national and international health inequalities and the promotion of public policy designed to influence corporate and individual behaviour. There is an integral assumption that the private sector tends to produce the problems and the public and professional sectors have a capacity and duty to produce solutions.

NPH literature acknowledges past achievements but asserts that their current proposals are qualitatively different. Ashton and Seymour began their seminal text with the statement: 'Until quite recently it has been a commonly held view that all improvements in health are the results of scientific medicine' (Ashton & Seymour, 1988: 1). This is worth considering in the light of the following:

> Medicine is no longer an affair of drugs – useful as these are in their place – and methods that were adopted by our barbarous ancestors when they called in the aid of the medicine man's incantations are nearly out of date. An organism badly born and badly bred, always placed under unwholesome conditions and slowly saturated with disease, finally breaks down and is brought to the doctor to be drugged into health: it is a sorry task for medical science, and, what is of much more consequence, it involves fearful expense, not merely to the individual but to all those with whom he comes into contact, expense of money, expense of happiness, expense of life. The key word of our modern methods is not cure but prevention, and while this task is more complex it is also far easier. It is to a gigantic system of healthy living, and by a perpetual avoidance of the very beginnings of evil, that our medical science is now leading us.

But for a verbal archaism or two this might serve as a current manifesto for the Public Health Alliance but in fact it comes from *The Nationalisation of Health* by Havelock Ellis, published in 1892 (Ellis, 1892: 18). It clearly goes beyond the older nineteenth century public health agenda. Ellis's means were just as striking as his ends: the pursuit of health demanded 'the nationalisation of health', the centralisation of all health activities in a state scheme, the establishment of school medical and dental services, better factory inspection to tackle industrial diseases and the appointment of full time Medical Officers of Health. His notion of the 'modern' health professional would please WHO. They would:

> … not to seek to pull out with spasmodic effort the mangled wretches who float down to the sea in a great torrent of disease and misery, but to help to maintain the dykes which protect us against the sources of disease and misery.

Doctors would be employees of the state and capable of imposing 'rational social organisation and rational individual behaviour' (Ellis, 1892: 240–241). When Ellis returned to this subject in 1913 in *The Task of Social Hygiene* (Ellis, 1913) he expressed his contempt for National Health Insurance that had been introduced just two years before he wrote. His reason was the same as that of Beatrice Webb; under the insurance principle 'the state gets nothing for its money in the way of conduct'(MacKenzie, 1984: 118), In current terms, insurance empowered the recipient, and the state gained no capacity to manipulate the recipient's behaviour (Nottingham, 1999: 173–181).

My intention is not to dismiss NPH on the basis of its antecedents. What however, such examples should suggest is that much of the NPH agenda has been understood and articulated over many years, but, for whatever reason, has failed to attract the support of policy makers.

So, to refine the question, how do we explain why an active, preventive, collective approach to population health, well understood and widely articulated, sat on the periphery of policy for a century and then took centre stage? Berridge suggests four 'milestones' in the recent recovery: the impact of the Acheson Report of 1988 on public health medicine, the rise of 'evidence based medicine', new ideas about health promotion imported from the international sector, and the movement for multi disciplinary public health in the 1990s (Berridge, 2006: xxi) and these can serve as useful clues.

Policy transfer was obviously one important factor. The fact that several industrialised countries, notably the USA and Canada, adopted strategies aimed at reducing heart disease, cancers and accidents during the 1970s and the World Health Organisation (WHO) issued the Alma Ata Declaration in 1978 and adopted Health for All (WHO, 1981) brought encouragement for British public health campaigners in their lowest moments. Such developments were also much welcomed and discussed by leaders in other British health professions, notably nursing, ever on the look out for something that might rescue them from the constraints of the Bevan/BMA doctor led service (Hart, 2004).

It is also necessary to allow for the impact of NPH supporters themselves. Theirs has been a persistent campaign with a number of professional and institutional foci, sometimes prestigious such as the Public Health Faculty of the Royal College of Physicians, and has included university departments, research units, ad hoc campaigns like Action on Smoking and Health, long term campaigning groups such as the Socialist Medical Association and cross disciplinary groups such as the Public Health Alliance as well as units of international and national government. Its methods have also been of a hybrid character. The binding agent is the cause, exemplified in core texts such as the Black Report. The discussion at the recent Wellcome witness seminar brought this complexity. Groups identified as having been significant included the National Perinatal Epidemiology Unit in Oxford the medical sociology section of the British Sociological Association (Berridge, 2006: 44–7) and particular courses at Universities such as 'the MSc in social medicine [...] at the London School of Hygiene and Tropical Medicine'. David Player, used the Health Education Unit of the *Scottish Office* in the 1980s to fund lectureships and chairs in Scottish universities with the intention 'to establish health education as a profession' (Nottingham, 2000: 74–5). The Society for Social Medicine was seen as an important multidisciplinary network (Berridge, 2006: 122). Such multidisciplinary tendencies were strengthened during the 1980s and 1990s with the NHS Research and Development Initiative. Occupational groups such as environmental health officers and specialists in occupational health were seen as critical in the breakdown of medical exclusivity (Berridge, 2006: 58–9). Others cited the Society of Health Education, health promotion officers, the statisticians group of the Royal College of

Physicians, community development workers, and radical health visitors. Individuals were invariably members of more than one group and an organisation such as the Public Health Alliance was crucial in binding individuals to the wider cause when they became drawn into particular campaigns (Berridge, 2006: 136; Macfarlane, 1999).

Some professions, such as environmental health officers, were always natural supporters, but most health professions had sections or groups of individuals who became enthusiasts. Individual doctors, often holding important official appointments, took leading positions in cause groups and campaigns. NPH had an even greater influence in the insecure health professions, that is professions with status difficulties, such as health visitors, midwives and nurses (Nottingham, 2007). For nursing leaders from the 1970s onwards NPH ideals and the 'social model' offered a welcome distraction from domestic frustrations, a sense of higher professional purpose and connections with international health agencies. The following extract captures the tone perfectly:

> Nurses the world over need to influence the political agenda in order to challenge the current inequitable access to health and health care resources, economic impoverishment, and unsafe physical surroundings that threaten the health and well-being of countless people. (Maslin-Prothero, 2002: 108–117)

However, while NPH ideas could have attained their present pre-eminence without this wave of activity it does not adequately explain the rise. Baggott has pointed out that NPH draws support from across the political spectrum but the unifying sentiments of campaigners were always egalitarian, socialist, rationalistic, statist, with a scepticism of, if not downright hostility towards market principles (Berridge, 2006: 38–42). And yet it was in the Thatcher era that current developments began. While Thatcher's ministers were anything but natural supporters of NPH, they were faced with events, such as salmonella in eggs, CJD, and most importantly the rise of AIDS, which persuaded them that some action of this sort was unavoidable (Berridge, 1996). Similarly there were inescapable pressures to take action on smoking and drug abuse. Certain aspects of the NPH agenda such as health inequalities, remained taboo, but when the Major government finally introduced public health white papers in 1992, *Health of the Nation* and *Scotland's Health A Challenge to us all*, it accepted targets for reducing heart disease and cancers and at least acknowledged 'health variations' that would have to be addressed. Although New Labour politicians in both England and Scotland have been much more explicit in their acceptance of public health perspectives, similar reasoning still applies. The idealistic rhetoric of NPH is incorporated into policy pronouncements, health inequalities are explicitly deplored but re-distributive solutions, favoured by NPH campaigners, are ignored. The aspects of NPH that seem to exercise most appeal to New Labour ministers are those which fit most readily with the New Public Management (NPM) agenda. A management driven service requires targets and NPH is ideally equipped to provide these for organisations, professionals and individuals. Moreover the imposition of overall targets and the assumption of a common purpose provides a framework for joint working and the erosion of demarcation lines between professions. Overall a combination of NPM and a selection of NPH measures seems to promise that better control over the NHS that politicians and mangers have sought since the Griffiths Report of 1983 and a way of coping with the recurring problems of health politics outlined above. NPH is taken up when it serves other requirements and even then is a highly selective way.

Outcomes

What then will be the likely results of the current move to apply NPH doctrines to the constitution of the health care state? One safe prediction is that they are unlikely to be what its advocates want. The discipline of politics has few rules but one dismal, inescapable one is that of unforeseen consequences. Rational plans are rarely adopted in their entirety and the results never correspond with their advocates' intentions.

Before going further it is helpful to consider some of the arguments of the opponents of NPH. The opposition cannot be categorised on any simple left/right continuum but at the core are a set of libertarian objections. The scourge of the professions, Ivan Illich (1977) was an early contributor. For Illich NPH was driven by the illegitimate ambition by doctors to extend their authority into different areas of life. Peter Berger (Berger, 1991) offered a more refined critique, complaining that NPH campaigns were disproportionate to the problems: 'The diseases that remain and kill, cancers and heart disease, are largely diseases of comparatively old age. Though they are responsible for loss of lots of lives, they are not responsible for the loss of many years of life' (Berger, 1991: 9). Berger disliked the fervour of NPH advocates suggesting it represented the transfer of religious values into the secular zone (Berger, 1991: 30). Irving Krystol saw behind NPH the machinations of a power hungry 'new class', imbued with a 'collectivist and statist' ideology, that seized on public health when denied access to power by conventional means; NPH 'spreads in spite of the political character' of governments (Berger, 1991: 40). Robert Browning detected an elite so determined to force their love on the unfortunate that when the unfortunate rejected their advances, "They set about building public policy apparatuses … to force people to take the medicine they had chosen to refuse' (Berger, 1991: 33). Browning particularly disliked that multi disciplinary nature of NPH; '… it is increasingly doctors of economics, sociology and politics rather than medicine who are to the fore in determining health policy' (Berger, 1991: 34). A similar point was developed by Fischer. NPH involved experts striving to usurp the power that was the legitimate preserve of elected politicians and health professionals (Fischer, 1990). Fischer F (1990), *Technocracy and the Politics of Expertise* Sage Digby Anderson argued that NPH downgraded personal and parental choice in favour of blanket regulation. Health education 'which places the emphasis on helping the individual to make responsible decisions' was permissible but not 'the new politicised health-activism or health promotion which involves activists and governments taking mass level decisions for different individuals and imposing mass solutions' (Berger, 1991: 40). For Skrabenek (1994) NPH represented the death of humane medicine. Health became a state ideology and granted too much authority to the state and the medical profession to interfere in the lives of individuals. Skrabenek (1994) Petersen and

Lupton (1996) provided the classical statement of the Foucaultian opposition: 'The new public health can be seen as but the most recent of a series of regimes of power and knowledge that are orientated to the regulation and surveillance of individual bodies and the social body as whole.' It 'provided opportunities for moral regulation making individuals more self regulating and productive in order to serve societies broader needs.' Castel (1991) similarly, saw NPH as driven by politicians themselves searching for a plan of 'governmentality' 'appropriate to the needs of advanced industrial societies'. Michael Fitzpatrick, writing as a family doctor, complained that NPH turned the doctor into a regulator and threatened his relationship with his patients. Moreover, it advanced the 'erosion of the boundaries between the public and the private spheres is one of the most ominous trends in modern society' (Fitzpatrick, 2001: 172).

The critics disagree as to whether it was the state, the social scientists or the doctors themselves who are the real villains, but their arguments do deal with the considerations that propel the guardians of the health care state in a NPH direction. Yet for anyone not inclined to see 'social control' in all its manifestations as irretrievably evil and unnecessary many of their arguments are ultimately unsatisfactory. NPH may, almost certainly does, appeal to politicians as plan of 'governmentality' appropriate to the needs of advanced industrial societies (Castel, 1991) but this is no reason to disapprove of it. Firstly, the conspiratorial assumption behind such statements is surely exaggerated. If nothing else they attribute far too much unfettered competence to the politicians. If we now have a 'strategy' it has emerged from the power-broking between professionals, health ministers, finance ministers, media and the public, and the relentless pressure of 'events'. Secondly, it is difficult to see something automatically reprehensible in the aspiration to take up elements of NPH. Neither politicians nor professionals have the luxury of disengagement. Working solutions have to be found and it is quixotic to assume that these can be achieved in ways that satisfy all requirements. Another criticism that can be raised against such arguments, Anderson excepted, is that they offer no guidance of how we might distinguish between interventions which are permissible and those that are not. Moreover there is no real dialogue. Neither pro nor anti camp descend from Olympian fundamentals. Neither, suggest a means of discussing the implications of NPH doctrines on the clinical encounter, the 'negotiated order' between professional and patient.

The politicians, to repeat, did not seize on NPH out of intellectual conviction. They do not embrace it in its entirety. The process is essentially similar to the one that persuaded nineteenth century politicians that the difficulties of a qualified incorporation of public health approaches were less than those associated with not doing so. The heightened risks of an increasingly interdependent society indicated that tolerable order could not be maintained without this new means of social governance (De Swaan, 1988). The process of adding NPH measures to the existing means of governance is not in essence very different. And similarly, the increased reliance on international health agencies does represent idealism but the practical recognition that the security of the domestic society can only protected by attention to the health of populations elsewhere.

Opponents tend to focus on the more extreme statements by NPH enthusiasts such as that by Montgomery who recently complained of 'many things public health doctors wanted to do in the interests of public health but were unable to do' and argued that 'some of our old assumptions on what the state should or should not do are inappropriate.' Examples suggested were greater controls over alcohol consumption and compulsory MMR vaccination. But he also raised the question of 'the extent to which people who decide to behave in ways that harm their health should be entitled to free treatment' (Day, 2006).

However, those that find this last idea troublesome can console themselves with the thought that it is unlikely to be translated into policy in pure form. In the first place citizens do not regard NHS treatment as free and its withdrawal will always be highly controversial in practice. In health politics we know, the publicity surrounding hard cases usually subverts policy. Similarly we can ask, would any politician have thought it possible to defend compulsory MMR vaccination at the height of the recent public anxieties? Moreover the most recalcitrant sections of the population in health behaviour are usually the poorest, so the application of such a policy would appear to threaten the health inequalities aspirations of NPH enthusiasts themselves. Although Patricia Hewitt grabs headlines with support for doctors who deny surgery to patients who smoke or are overweight, a close reading of statements shows denial is based on the grounds that such behaviours compromise the effectiveness of the treatment. Moreover, she added, 'it would be dreadful to deny treatment on the grounds that patients were to blame for their condition' (*Daily Telegraph*, 12 February 2007). It is also important to remember that the smoking bans were not brought in when it became widely accepted that smoking was dangerous for individual smokers but when smokers had become a minority and the majority wanted smoke-free public places.

In imagining consequences of the new policies it is always important to remember that other aspects of the relationship between states, professionals and their patients remain the same. The 'Republic of Choice' will not dissolve on contact with NHP. (Friedman, 1990), and in this republic there is permanent conflict between the ethos of public health campaigners and the popular culture of individualism, consumerism and choice. Even if we feel states or professionals are harbouring illegitimate aspirations to control populations it is unlikely that they would get away with it.

However, although the fears of the anti NPH campaigners may be exaggerated there are two substantial difficulties with the application of NPH inspired policies. Both concern the relationship between health professionals and patients and both threaten the very aims that NPH supporters hold dearest. The first is the suspicion that the more directional role of health professionals, inspired by NPH policies and reinforced by the demands of NPM, will be far more disruptive of their relationships with one type of patient than another. The many patients who are already inclined to take health concerns into account in making choices about eating or exercise may accept, even welcome, a higher degree of intrusion. There is however another category of patient. If their visits to the doctor become a matter of tests that reveal past offences and instructions to alter their current behaviour there is a risk that they will avoid health care professionals wherever possible. As many such patients are likely to be the ones who provide the disturbing statistics on premature death such measures could actually increase health inequalities.

The second, related, concern is the propensity of the combinations of NPH and NPM to reduce the effectiveness of health care professionals. We are well aware that some groups of professionals, social workers for instance, experience far greater difficulties in their encounter with clients that others. It takes no great leap of the imagination to see that these differences are related to the client's perceptions of the encounter. Roughly the professional who is seen to be responding to a client's stated need has a far better chance of establishing a productive relationship with the client than one seen to be bearing an agenda. One should never underestimate the capacity of professionals to make 'street level' adjustments to soften the official instructions they work under, but the tendency of NPH/NPM policies promises to make this more difficult. An A&E nurse under the injunction to check for evidence of abuse or malnutrition in children, a dentist compelled to check for alcohol abuse in his patient's mouth, a community nurse on the look out for evidence of domestic violence, or any health professional warning patients that treatment depends upon behaviour, are all in a different position to the one professional instincts might decree. The new rules, in short, threaten the 'negotiated order' between client and professional, and hence the effectiveness of those who maintain contacts between official and unofficial worlds. The impact, again, could be greatest on the groups that give the most cause for concern.

The most troublesome part of the current situation is the lack of nuanced political debate. NPH campaigners acknowledge the political nature of their prescriptions. Yet they see politics as no more than a mechanism for transferring their insights into practice. The opposition focuses too much on the aspiration of enthusiasts, ignores the complexities of application, and recommends, by implication, a return to a status quo that is not regarded as workable by either the medical profession or the politicians. A more productive debate might well begin with a return to that lively public discourse around state action and individual rights that took place in the last decades of the nineteenth century. The current dialogue of the deaf could only be improved if we thought, for instance, in terms of self and other regarding actions, and negative and positive definitions of liberty. Mill, Green and Hobhouse won't solve current difficulties but would get us beyond naive zero sum arguments. Harris's insight that that late nineteenth century debate on state powers took place at a time when collectivism and individualism were both on the rise, might prove particularly useful (Harris, 1994).

So, in conclusion, it is not difficult to identify the pressures that have pushed the Scottish Executive in this direction. It seems to justify the devolution arrangements, it might appear to rectify the socialist deficit in other parts of New Labour policy, and, as a low cost, high visibility policy, might deflect attention from the grind of mainstream health politics. Moreover in combination with NPM it offers some prospect of establishing some greater degree of control over this problematical mainstream. It should not however be conceptualised as a policy which will eliminate the rights of individuals, but rather as a means of balancing the requirements of an increasingly demanding and ever less deferential public with the need to moderate the rise in health budgets and attain some control over the working of the NHS. The Bevan/BMA Health Service, was a rough and ready means of balancing contradictory requirements. The 'medical model' had its clinical limitations but it was workable politically. However it went into decline, not least because the doctors, on whom it rested, no longer felt able to discharge their former responsibilities.

If the worst fears of the opponents of NPH seem unrealistic there are still potentially serious problems with the NPH/NPM model, particularly as it restructures the relationship between the professional and the patient. Doctors will experience new pressures but it is perhaps not necessary to worry over much about their capacity to cope. The new model will demand adjustment but the authority of the profession is so great and the state's need for its services so pressing, that it is reasonable to suppose that it can achieve a satisfactory settlement. It is more difficult to see a satisfactory outcome for the insecure professions in healthcare. The erosion of demarcation lines will bring welcome benefits but the acquisition of new agendas may make street level encounters with patients less comfortable. Ironically, the tendency of NPH may be to compromise the relationships on which the core aim of the policy, the aspiration to improve the health of the poorest and less engaged citizens, actually depends.

References

Ashton, J., and Seymour, H. (1988), *The New Public Health*, Open University Press Books, Milton Keynes.

Baggott, R. (2000), *Public Health: Policy and politics*, Palgrave Macmillan, Basingstoke.

Berger, P. (ed.) (1991), *Health, Lifestyle and Environment: Countering the Panic*, Social Affairs Unit/Manhattan Institute, London/New York.

Berridge, V. (1996), *AIDS in the UK: The making of policy 1981–1994*, Oxford University Press, Oxford.

Berridge, V., Christie, D.A. and Tansey, A.M. (2006), 'Public Health in the 1980s and 1990s: Decline and Rise', Transcript of a Witness Seminar, Wellcome Trust Centre for the History of Medicine at UCL, London, on 12 October 2004

Castel, R. (1991), 'From Dangerousness to Risk', in Burchell, G., Gordon, G., and Miller, P. (eds), *The Foucault Effect: Studies in Governmentality*, Harvester Wheatsheaf, Hemel Hemstead.

Cm 1986 (1992), *The Health of the Nation. A Consultative Document for Health in England*, HMSO, London.

Cmnd 289 (1988), *Public Health in England: The Report of the Committee of Inquiry into the Future Development of the Public Health Function* (Acheson Report) HMSO, London.

Cmnd 9716 (1986), Report of a committee of Inquiry into an Outbreak of Food Poisoning at Stanley Royd Hospital, Wakefield, HMSO, London.

Department of Health and Social Security (DHSS) (1980), *Inequalities in Health: The Black Report*, HMSO, London.

Day, M. (2006), *BMJ* **332**, 1176 (20 May).

De Swaan, A. (1988), *In Care of the State*, Polity Press, Cambridge.

DHSS (1983), *NHS Management Inquiry* (The Griffiths Management Report), London.

DHSS (1980), *Report of the Working Group on Inequalities in Health* (The Black report), DHSS, London.

DHSS (1986), 'Report of the Committee of Inquiry into an Outbreak of Food Poisoning at Stanley Royd Hospital', 'Stanley Royd Inquiry', Cm. 9716, HMSO, London.

Fitzpatrick, M. (2001), *The Tyranny of Health*, Routledge, London.

Friedman, L. (1990), *The Republic of Choice*, Harvard University Press, Cambridge Mass.

Harris, J. (1994), *Private Lives, Public Spirit: Britain 1870–1914*, Penguin, London.

Hart, C. (2004), *Nurses and Politics: The Impact of Power and Practice*, Palgrave, London.

Ellis, H. (1892), *The Nationalisation of Health*, T. Fisher Unwin, London.

Ellis, H. (1912), *The Task of Social Hygiene*, Constable, London.

Fischer, F. (1990), *Technocracy and the Politics of Expertise*, Sage, London.

H. M. Treasury (2004), *Securing Good Health for the Whole Population: Final report*, London.

Illich, I. (1977), *Limits to Medicine: Medical nemesis: The expropriation of health*, Penguin, Harmondsworth, New York.

Leck, I. (1996), 'The Society for Social Medicine, 1956–96', *Journal of Epidemiology and Community Health*, **50**, 177.

Petersen, A. and Lupton, D. (1996), *The New Public Health: Discourses, Knowledges and Strategies*, Sage, London.

Macfarlane, A. (1999), 'Lessons and laughs from the past: How the Health Group developed', *Radical Statistics*, **71**.

MacKenzie, N. and J. (1984), *The Diary of Beatrice Webb*, Vol.3 1905–1924, Virago and LSEPS, London.

Maslin-Prothero, S. and Masterson, A. (May 2002), 'Power, Politics and Nursing in the United Kingdom', *Policy Politics and Nursing Practice*, **3**(2) 108–117.

McKeown, T. (1976), *The Modern Rise of Population*, Edward Arnold, London.

NHS Management Inquiry Report (Griffths Report) (1983), DHSS, London.

NHS Scotland (2006), *Health in Scotland 2005*, Edinburgh.

Nottingham, C. (1999), *The Pursuit of Serenity: Havelock Ellis and the New Politics*, Amsterdam University Press, Amsterdam.

Nottingham, C. (ed.) (2000), *The NHS in Scotland: The Legacy of the Past and the Prospect of the Future*, Ashgate Publishing Ltd, Aldershot.

Nottingham, C. (December 2007), 'The Rise of the Insecure Professionals', *International Review of Social History*, (Forthcoming).

Scottish Executive (2000), 'Our National Health: A Plan for Action, A Plan for Change', *Scottish Executive*, Edinburgh.

Scottish Executive (2003), *Partnership for Care: Scotland's Health White Paper*, *Scottish Executive*, Edinburgh.

Scottish Office (1992), 'Scotland's health: A challenge to us all: a policy statement', *Scottish Office*, Edinburgh.

Skrabenek, P. (1994), The Death of Humane Medicine, Social Affairs Unit, London.

Stewart, J. (1999), *The Battle for Health. A Political History of the Socialist Medical Association, 1930–51*, Ashgate Publishing Ltd, Aldershot.

World Health Organization (WHO)/UNICEF (1978), Alma Ata, *Primary Health Care*, WHO, Geneva.

WHO (1981), *Global Strategy for Health for All by the Year 2000*, Geneva: WHO.

Chapter 10

Taking the Wait Off: An Examination of the Influence of Policy Networks in a Case where Local Policy was Formulated and Implemented, to Reduce Protracted Waiting for Orthopaedic Services

M-L. O'Driscoll

The existence of a gap between demand for and supply of health care services has posed a policy dilemma for United Kingdom (UK) Governments, since the start of the National Health Service (NHS). In the absence of infinite resources to meet an ever-growing demand for health care, a variety of strategies have been used to balance the equation. Amongst them is waiting, which has been described as rationing by delay (Klein, Day et al., 1996: 11–12, 2001: 45–46). From the patients' perspective, waiting for diagnosis or treatment of a health problem is frustrating. Delay in treatment can be distressing for patients and their carers and unsettling for the health professionals who have to deal with the physical and psycho-social consequences. Waiting is equally problematic when viewed from a political and policy perspective. In the UK, where the health service is publicly funded from general taxation, any suggestion that the public is not getting good value for money is politically sensitive. This has become increasingly the case over the last twenty-five years. As governments have become sensitised to waiting, it has come to be regarded as a measure of the success of their health policies (Bourn, 2001: 1–2; Bradshaw and Bradshaw, 2004: 40–41). Despite being a measure that is notoriously elusive and unreliable, both politicians and the media have come to believe in waiting as an indicator of adequate funding and efficiency in the health service (Bradshaw and Bradshaw, 2004: 40–41). Long waiting lists have come to 'embody bureaucracy, slowness and inconvenience' in health services (Bourn, 2001: 1–2). Unsurprisingly UK governments, whilst not discouraging its use as a rationing device in their battle to balance demand and supply, have tried a variety of approaches to bring waiting down to acceptable levels.

Devolving responsibility to Local Health Authorities (and more recently to NHS Trusts and then to Strategic Health Authorities), has been an approach adopted by government to manage demand and supply in the health service. Since the early

1990s, the above local health organisations have been charged with assessing the health needs of their local population and ensuring that resources are deployed efficiently to meet those needs (see the NHS and Community Care Act, 1990). In order to retain control over measures such as waiting, which are politically sensitive, the government has set targets against which the performance of local health service organisations can be gauged. Where these organisations have failed to achieve government targets, they have been required to develop and implement local policy solutions which are sensitive to the needs of their population. How local health service organisations work with local stakeholder groups to develop local policies, in response to national policies, has not been examined in great detail either by academics or by wider society. Greenaway, Smith et al. (1992: 3) have suggested that the media frequently covers the decisions made by the parliamentary elite, whilst ignoring what happens in local authorities, thereby hiding key elements of British government from public view. This seems to be the case for the management of local health service resources, including those affecting patient waiting.

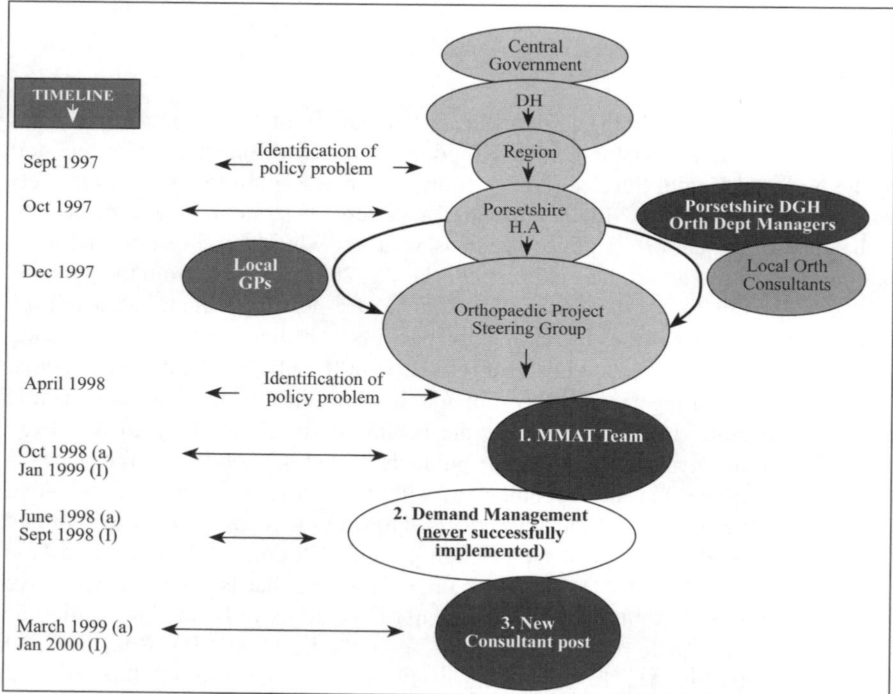

Figure 10.1 Diagram depicting the chronology of the events leading up to and including the policy implementation in the Porsetshire Case ((a) = Agreement to adopt policy preference and (I) = Policy Implemented)

This case study examines the decisions and actions of a group of health service managers and clinicians who were charged with resolving a local policy problem, which involved protracted waiting for orthopaedic services. It studies their interpretation of the national policy on waiting, and their re-formulation and implementation of that policy in the form of a local waiting list initiative. The case study specifically explores the influence of policy networks on the local policy processes and the policy outcomes. Figure 10.1 illustrates the networks and other organisations involved in the policy process and the chronology of policy formulation and implementation. The case being studied is located in a period between 1997 and 2000, in a part of the UK which will be referred to as 'Porsetshire'. The decision was taken to anonymise the area in which this case is located because the case study looks in detail at the motivations and behaviours of a number of key actors. It was therefore decided that these actors should be afforded the protection of anonymity in this and other publications.

Methods Adopted in this Case Study

The data that has been analysed in this policy case study was originally collected as part of a commissioned evaluation of the policy initiative developed in Porsetshire. The data comprised:

- Minutes of meetings of the group who formulated the Porsetshire waiting list initiative and oversaw its implementation.
- Documents tabled for discussion at the above meetings.
- Observations recorded during some of the above meetings.
- Interviews with key policy decision makers involved in the policy process.
- Interviews with members of the policy networks, seen to be at work in the policy process.

During the course of the original evaluation project, the researcher had secured the appropriate permissions for re-analysis of the above materials for a PhD study and subsequent publications.

For the case study presented here, a qualitative approach has been adopted in the analysis of the above documentary and interview materials. Both a 'top down' and a 'bottom up' approach have been deployed to select and analyse the data. The top down approach (Mason, 2002: 152–153) was used to identify the individuals and groups of agents involved in the policy process and to map the national and local policy structures (policy context) within which they were operating. The bottom up approach, adapted from that described by Strauss and Corbin (1998) and Charmaz (2000), was used to explore the concerns, issues and ideas circulating in the policy arena and their influence on the policy process. A narrative of the policy process that was constructed was set alongside a chronological story of the national health policies that informed the local policy-makers in Porsetshire. This narrative was further examined through a theoretical 'lens' that combined 'policy network theory' and 'ideas'. This lens, which is further explained below, permitted the identification of causal influences on the policy process and policy outcomes in the Porsetshire case.

The Rationale for the Theoretical Framework Deployed in this Case Study

The theoretical framework adopted for the study of the Porsetshire case was 'policy network theory'. The way in which this framework incorporated consideration of the role of 'ideas', in the study of policy formulation and implementation in Porsetshire, is depicted in Figure 10.2.

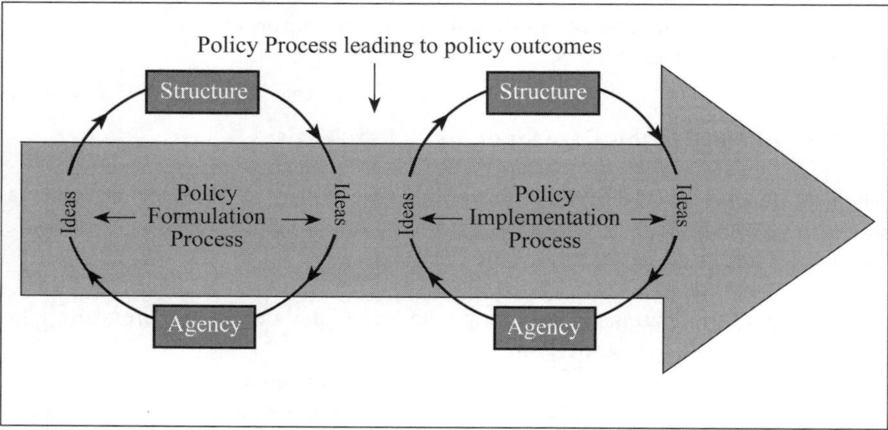

Figure 10.2 Diagram depicting the meta-theoretical thinking that underpins the study of policy formulation and implementation processes in the Porsetshire case

It is widely acknowledged that, in stable liberal democracies, policy is made in communities of policy actors, who operate within political institutions that interact to influence policy outcomes (John, 1998: 78–91; Marsh and Smith, 2000). Policy network theory offers a meso-level framework through which it is possible to study the influence of both structure and agency on policy outcomes (Marsh, 1998: 15; Rhodes and Marsh, 1992: 12; Rhodes, 1997: 29). Whilst acknowledging the influence of both, some proponents of policy network theory privilege structure over agency or vice versa. This study has opted, however, to scrutinise the iterative or dialectical relationship between structure and agents. It has sought to explore the informal as well as the formal associations that might have influenced policy decision-making, in a manner similar to that advocated by Marsh and Smith (2000). Furthermore, it has sought to understand the motivation for behaviours seen within and between policy networks. To achieve the latter, the decision was taken to actively examine 'ideas' circulating in policy networks and being represented by actors during the policy formulation and implementation processes in Porsetshire, in a manner similar to that described by Hay (2002: 213). In taking the above decision, ideas were deemed to have a crucial role in the critical explanation of the policy processes and policy outcomes in the Porsetshire case. Since it was perceived that actors could not have perfect knowledge of the world in which they operated, they were seen as having to 'interpret' that world. Ideas, in this study, were therefore regarded as 'a point of mediation between the actor and their environment' (op. cit: 211–212).

Policy Networks at Work in the Porsetshire Case

The policy network typology utilised in this case study was that developed by Rhodes (Rhodes and Marsh, 1992: 13; Rhodes, 1997: 38–39). This typology distinguishes between five different types of network:

1. Issue networks – loose networks comprising a large number of participants united, as their name suggests, by a focus on a particular issue.
2. Producer networks – characterised by their particular concerns with economic interests and their dependence on others for delivering goods and expertise.
3. Inter-governmental networks – expressing a wide range of interests across a range of services and having the ability to penetrate a variety of other networks.
4. Professional networks – expressing an interest in a particular profession.
5. Policy communities – described as a network but characterised by their highly restrictive membership and shared service delivery responsibilities.

This typology, more usually used in the analysis of national policies, was developed by Rhodes to permit examination of the influence of structures on policy processes and outcomes (Rhodes, 1997: 36). Although this case study was interested in the influence of both structures and agents, Rhodes' typology was valued for the number of different networks it described and the detail in which each type was described. Both of these attributes eased the identification of networks in the Porsetshire case and so assisted the analysis of their influence.

The networks seen to influence the local orthopaedic waiting policy, in Porsetshire, were:

(a) A local orthopaedic steering group, comprising managers and senior clinicians, who took on policy responsibility for the Porsetshire waiting list problem, in a manner similar to that seen in a policy community.
(b) A producer network of health service managers, comprising managers from the Porsetshire Health Authority and managers from the orthopaedic department in the Porsetshire District General Hospital (DGH).
(c) A professional network of General practitioners.
(d) A professional network of orthopaedic consultant surgeons.
(e) A group of non-medical clinicians involved in the management of patients with orthopaedic conditions.
(f) Patients and their carers who had an interest in seeing orthopaedic waiting times reduced.

These networks and groups of actors, evident in the Porsetshire policy arena, are depicted in Figure 10.3 below.

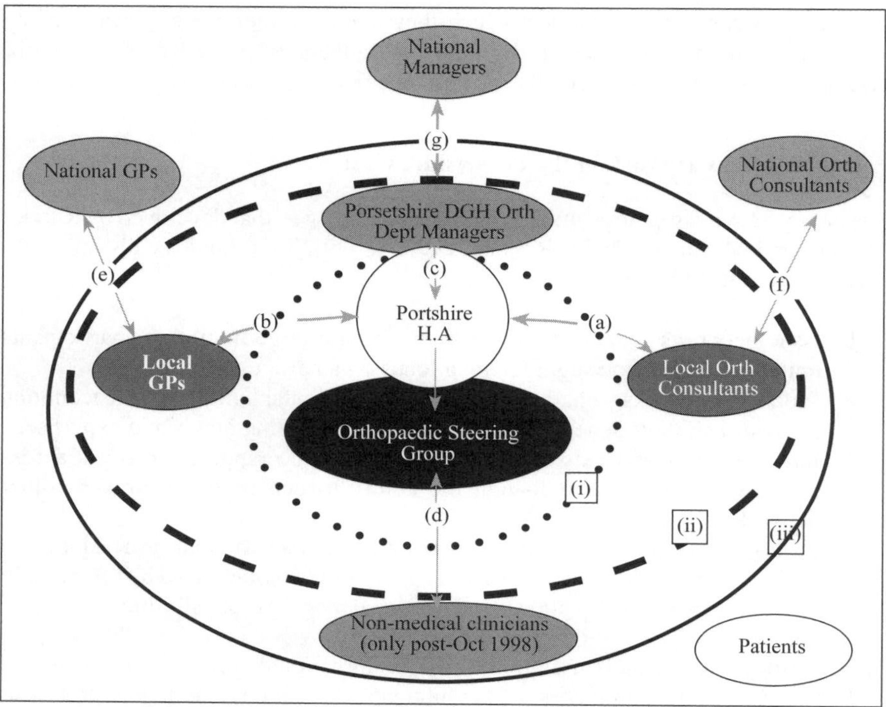

Figure 10.3 Diagram depicting the Orthopaedic Steering Group and the extent to which it could be penetrated by policy networks wishing to influence the Porsetshire policy process

The relationships between the orthopaedic steering group, who formulated the Porsetshire policy for the management of waiting for orthopaedic services, and the other local networks/groups are described in Figure 10.3 through the use of arrows ((a) to (g)) and concentric lines (i to iii). Arrows (a) to (d) indicate the routes through which network representatives were invited to join the orthopaedic steering group. Arrows (e) to (g) indicate the relationships that local networks maintained with their peers nationally. The concentric lines indicate the extent to which each of the local networks or groups were able to penetrate the local policy-making process and influence policy formulation and implementation. The degree to which a network/group was excluded from the policy process is represented in terms of their distance from the centre of the diagram. The contributions of key networks to policy process will be explored in the narratives below. It is however noted that patients were at no time invited to participate in the policy process. Furthermore, non-medical clinicians were only invited to participate in the process after October 1998, once it was decided that their professions were needed as part of the policy solution and once most decisions had been taken. Alas, discussion of the exclusion of these two groups of stakeholders is beyond the scope of this chapter.

Study of the data collected via observation of meetings, minutes of steering group meetings and interviews with actors in the policy arena, revealed that the networks involved in the policy process each had their own set of interests and concerns. These are outlined in Table 10.1. The extent to which the concerns of these networks influenced policy formulation and implementation will be explored in the narrative of the policy process, presented below.

Table 10.1 Table listing the key concerns of the networks most actively involved in the Porsetshire policy formulation process

Management	GPs	Consultants
Meeting targets and staying 'on budget'	Feeling that their referral practices are viewed as the cause of waiting	Feeling overwhelmed by their workload
Being seen as responsive (and original)	Feeling under pressure from patients to refer	Feeling that others view them as responsible for waiting
Being seen as fair to all parties	Lamenting the loss of orthopaedic in-service training for GPs	
	Wanting efficient use of 'their' money	

Through informal discussions with the researcher and comments made at meetings, the managers revealed themselves to be particularly concerned about finance for their services and about achieving targets. One of the Porsetshire Health Authority managers commented *come hell or high water we need to balance our books so something needs to be sorted out* (respondent P P2,17). Their concern about targets was linked to the issue of finance, insofar as they were in part motivated by possible financial penalties if targets were not met. However, they were also concerned with ensuring provision of the best patient care possible: *It's our duty to make sure that standards don't slip on our watch* (respondent W W1,79).

Where they fell short of the targets set, they were keen to be seen as responsive and indeed innovative in their efforts. One of the Porsetshire Health authority managers explained to the researcher that *if we can devise an effective solution to this one then we will lead the way for others who are dogged by the same problem [protracted orthopaedic waiting lists]* (respondent W FNW1,55). The same respondent also explained the importance of any policy solution being seen as fair – *it [any waiting list solution devised] must not be perceived as favouring the GPs or favouring the Hospital* (respondent W FNW1,202).

From interviews and comments in meetings, the GPs main concern was about the pressures on them to act as gate keepers to the waiting list. However, they were also concerned about ensuring that money that followed the patient was spent effectively on high quality patient services. As gate keepers GPs felt that they were under pressure, sometimes undue pressure, from patients to refer:

> they will either go and see someone else within the practice who says 'yes', or cause a stink or complain so vociferously that it would have been a lot quicker, for the service as a whole, to give them the second opinion that they requested in the first place. (respondent A A1,107).

At the same time GPs felt under pressure from hospital clinicians and managers, who they believed expected them to hold back a *flood-tide of demand* (respondent H H1,372). The majority of GPs interviewed talked about how they had valued in-service training that had existed prior to the institution of the internal market. They felt that this had not only offered them a way of maintaining clinical currency in the field of orthopaedics, but had also served as a space in which they could give voice to their concerns about waiting. In so doing they felt that they and their consultant colleagues had shared the responsibility for waiting lists in a way that they no longer did.

In addition to the pressures of gate keeping, GP interviews revealed a particular concern about the money they managed, in their capacity as fundholders (pre 1998) and as commissioners of services through their Primary Care Groups (post 1998). Every GP interviewed for the study commented on this matter in some way. One summed up the views of others very succinctly:

> We have a duty … I'm the patients' advocate and I'm obliged to ensure that I spend money wisely on their care. It really ticks me off when I see the hospital wasting money through inefficiencies, lost notes, appointment letters going astray, operating theatres sitting unused (respondent M M2,55).

The concerns of the orthopaedic consultants, revealed in interviews and meetings, were primarily about the extent to which they felt overworked and indeed overwhelmed when the waiting list was longer than that which targets prescribed. This feeling was to some extent compounded by a conviction that hospital managers, GPs and the public all viewed them as being the source of the waiting list problem, when they perceived the problem to be a whole systems one. One consultant vividly described the angst that he felt regarding the state of his waiting list:

> I need to get my waiting list down. The thing that bugs me is the waiting list, the letters, the constant pressure from everybody, the patients, administration, doctors to do surgery. That is what fills my day. That has got to be got down and the only way to do it is to do more operating. It is a laughable analogy. The water is coming in I am turning the taps off as much as I can, but everybody else wants to turn the taps on. The government just turn the tap on when it wants to so like this eighteen to fifteen month thing, boom, in comes a whole heap of water. So you have got to make the plughole bigger and the only way to do that is to do more operating so therefore I have got to have more theatre lists and everything that goes with that and outpatients can stay the same until it is in balance. And

> then you need a lot more orthopaedic surgeons to keep it all in balance because when you decrease the outpatient waiting time, patients will come out of the woodwork and keep coming (respondent B B1,99).

A number of consultants interviewed, when discussing the burden they felt from their waiting list, made reference to patients awaiting elective joint replacements. They regarded this group of patients as one for whom disability and distress could increase markedly if they were required to wait for treatment.

The next two sections will provide a chronological narrative of Porsetshire policy formulation and implementation and will expose the extent to which the above network concerns, network structures and national policy context influenced those processes.

A Chronological Narrative: The Porsetshire Policy Formulation Process (Presented Alongside the National Policy Context)

At the start of the time in which the Porsetshire case study is located, the Blair Labour Government had been recently elected. The government had come to power on 2 May 1997, with a majority of 179, on a mandate to reduce NHS waiting by 100K nationally. In the immediate aftermath of their election, the Labour party continued to pledge that they would secure £300 million for health, a large proportion of which would be directed towards tackling waiting (Baker, 2000: 4). However, despite having outlined its policy on health two years earlier, the party took seven months to publish its first policy document. In the absence of new policies emerging from the Labour government, the NHS continued to operate under policies generated by the previous Conservative government. Particular influences on the NHS culture of the time were:

(a) the 'Health of the Nation' White Paper – which had introduced health service targets and performance monitoring;
(b) the 1995 version of 'The Patients Charter' – which had made a commitment that patients requiring hip or knee surgery should receive treatment within 18 months and that 9 out of 10 patients awaiting outpatient appointments should be seen within 13 weeks (and everyone should be seen within 26 weeks).

In the September of 1997, four months after the Labour party election victory, the Regional Health Authority (RHA), responsible for Porsetshire and adjacent areas, identified that within its region 2532 patients were waiting for orthopaedic treatment on outpatient waiting lists. Of those waiting, 225 patients (8.89 per cent) had waited between 9 and 11 months and 186 patients (7.4 per cent) had waited longer than 12 months. 79.5 per cent of those waiting longer than 12 months were waiting in Porsetshire. The dimensions of the waiting problem in Porsetshire were clearly at odds with the government's stated target, whereby outpatients were to be seen within 13 weeks. Moreover, the RHA recognised that there had been a problem in Porsetshire for some years, which had not been effectively addressed. In October of 1997, the RHA asked the Porsetshire Health Authority to look into the matter urgently.

As 1997 drew to a close, a more radical vision for the NHS had begun to emerge from national government. A number of policy documents introduced new imperatives into the NHS culture and seemed to influence the approach adopted by local managers and clinicians in Porsetshire who were charged with tackling the waiting problem:

- In December 1997, the 'The New NHS: Modern. Dependable' white paper was published (Secretary of State for Health 1997). This paper made some minimal reference to waiting insofar as it emphasised the importance of prompt, high-quality care, but it did not set any new targets. It did, however, present some other important value statements and policy proposals. It emphasised the importance of partnership working and collaboration within the NHS. It introduced National Service Frameworks, which were intended to bring together best evidence of clinical effectiveness and cost effectiveness. It also laid the foundations for a revised structure of the NHS, introducing Primary Care Groups (PCGs) and replaced GP fund holding with PCG commissioning. Finally, it charged Health Authorities with assessing the needs of their population and distributing resources for the services required accordingly.
- In June 1998 'A first Class Service' (Secretary of State for Health 1998) was published. This emphasised the importance of quality in health care provision (including reducing waiting). It also valued evidence based practice and introduced new organisations charged with ensuring that NHS practice was evidence based (i.e. CHI and NICE).

In Porsetshire, as the end of 1997 approached, the Local Health Authority (LHA) had identified that 5000 referrals were being made annually from primary care. This was double the hospital capacity of 2500 appointments for orthopaedic specialists. Furthermore, analysis of the Porsetshire orthopaedic waiting list identified that many of the patients being referred did not, in fact, require the services of an orthopaedic surgeon. In the spirit of partnership working and collaboration, called for in the 'The New NHS: Modern. Dependable' white paper, the LHA looked for a policy solution that involved not only hospital based provider services but also community based gatekeepers and commissioners of services. They decided upon the introduction of a demand management strategy coupled with a concerted initiative or surgical "blitz" to reduce the number of patients on the waiting list. Their plan was based upon a strategy that they had heard about through their connection to other managers across the UK (see arrow (g) in Figure 10.3). The strategy had recently been employed in both Armagh and in Kings Lynn. The demand management element of the policy involved permitting GPs access to only a limited number of slots into which they could refer patients each year. At the time at which the LHA was proposing adopting the above strategy, it was regarded as novel and was widely believed to have proved successful at slowing the flow of referrals to waiting lists and encouraging hospital surgeons to 'get on top' of their waiting lists.

The LHA recognised that if it were to successfully implement its proposed policy of demand management, it needed the co-operation of local clinicians and managers. Furthermore it recognised that in working collaboratively with local clinicians from primary and secondary care, it would be seen to embrace national policy. In December 1997, it convened a meeting and invited representatives of the following networks to attend:

- Porsetshire orthopaedic consultants;
- General Practitioners (GPs) from the local, newly formed, PCGs; and
- Managers responsible for the delivery of orthopaedic services at the Porsetshire District General Hospital (see arrows (a) to (c) in Figure 10.3).

The LHA was not prepared for what happened next. At the above meeting, rather than approving the proposed local policy and agreeing to help implement it, the consultants and GPs collaborated in challenging it. Perhaps united by their shared professional identities, the GPs' and consultants' aggressive stance against the managers culminated in them forming a steering group, in which they could consider a range of other policy options that might replace or, at the very least complement, the LHA's policy proposal. Effectively the doctors had wrestled the policy formulation responsibilities out of the hands of the LHA and had bestowed them on a group which included representatives from GP, consultant and manager networks. Where the LHA might previously have been regarded as a local-level policy community, that status was re-assigned to the newly formed steering group. It is a moot point whether the LHA could have resisted this move, given their dependence on the doctors for later implementation of their proposed waiting list initiative.

In a period between December 1997 and April 1998 the new steering group (or new local policy community) met regularly (every 4–6 weeks). The minutes of their meetings recorded that a large number of policy proposals were suggested and considered by the group. Table 10.2 lists the various policies proposed and the network representatives who made each of the suggestions. From this table it is possible to see how both the national policy context and the various networks' concerns informed the list of policy proposals, from which the steering group could select a policy.

However, achieving agreement upon which of the above proposals should be adopted proved challenging. Despite pressure from the RHA, network representatives within the steering group fiercely defended their own network's interests and refused to compromise regarding the needs and wants of the other networks. Table 10.3 details the preferences for each of the policy options held by the managers, GPs and consultants in the spring of 1998.

Table 10.2 Table listing potential policy solutions (policy options) that were proposed by the various networks involved in the policy process between December 1997 and April 1998

Proposed policy solution	Group
Development of a **paramedic clinic** to deal with those patients on the waiting list who did not need surgery, but who did have a significant clinical problem, and so could not simply be discharged. This proposal was based on a similar local initiative, which had been recently developed by fellow local consultants, to manage patients with spinal problems. At the time that it was suggested consultants and GPs had observed it to be very effective at reducing waits for a spinal surgery consultation.	Consultants and GPs
Development of an **education programme** for GPs and surgeons to improve handling of referrals by both groups. This proposal seems closely linked to the GP network's desire to re-establish orthopaedic in-service training.	GP
Review of an in-service document, produced in 1993, which had recommended **addressing a number of service inefficiencies**, some of which had still not been addressed.	LHA
Focusing all efforts on clearing the waiting list of elective joint replacement patients via a surgical **'blitz'**. This proposal appears linked to elective joint replacement patients being one of the groups that particularly increased the sense of burden, felt by consultants regarding their waiting lists.	Consultants
Appointment of a **ninth consultant** orthopaedic surgeon. This proposal clearly reflects the consultants' desire to ease their workload and the burden they perceived in relation to the existing waiting list.	Consultants
Working to ensure maximum **efficiency** in the use of theatres. This proposal clearly reflects GPs concern to see 'their' money spent wisely.	GPs
Doing nothing until money was provided from government for an initiative.	Consultants
Reconsidering the merits of the **demand management** project that had been proposed by the Local Health Authority at the end of 1997. This proposal clearly emerged from a pool of policy ideas regarding approaches to waiting, circulating amongst a national network of managers.	LHA

The deadlock was only overcome in April 1998, following the Chancellor of the Exchequer's announcement of an increase in the NHS budget (Harrison and Appleby 2005, p, 8). This announcement was accompanied by a clear indication that the government was now expecting NHS targets, including those on waiting, to be met (ibid.). With the promise of access to tangible funds, the steering group overcame their differences. The steering group recognised that they were most likely to win future funding if they could agree upon and implement some sort of initiative to address local waiting. Despite the GPs reservations about the demand management proposal, it was recognised as an innovative approach and so, desirable. Moreover its adoption was thought to be supported by evidence of its success, from the Armagh and Kings Lynn projects, and so seen to conform to the national policy requirement for NHS evidence-based practice. By the summer of 1998 it had been tentatively agreed that this approach should be adopted and should be implemented from September 1998.

Table 10.3 Table displaying the Porsetshire policy networks policy preferences

Management	GPs	Consultants
Pro demand management slots	Had experienced little long term benefit from surgical "blitz" on waiting lists.	No objection to demand management slots
No objection to paramedic clinic	**Pro paramedic clinic**	**Aggressively pro ninth consultant**
No objection to ninth consultant	**Increasingly fiercely anti demand management slots**	**Pro paramedic clinic**
	No objection ninth Consultant	

In the autumn of 1998, the steering group had also agreed to adopt the paramedic clinic proposal and had duly invited representatives from the local orthopaedic nurse and physiotherapy communities to join the steering group to plan such a clinic (see arrow (d) in Figure 10.3). Both GPs and consultants actively supported the idea and it was seen as relatively inexpensive to set up. Moreover it was seen as source of relief for GPs who might find themselves managing a larger burden of patients in the community as a result of demand management.

Agreement on the third and final element of the Porsetshire waiting list initiative to be adopted was secured in the spring of 1999. Aware of the £20 million for new theatres and diagnostic equipment released in February 1999 and perhaps aware of the promise of £30 million to be released in the summer as a 'performance fund' intended to support a reduction in waiting, the steering group agreed to bid for funds to appoint a ninth consultant. They constructed a case stating that managers, GPs and consultants in Porsetshire had collaborated to develop an innovative and evidence-based initiative.

Their strategic spinning of the truth, which emphasised their responsiveness, cross-sector collaboration, innovation and the use of evidence, was eventually rewarded in the autumn of 1999 by the award of funding for a new consultant appointment.

A Chronological Narrative: The Porsetshire Policy Implementation Process (Presented Alongside the National Policy Context)

During the policy implementation phase in Porsetshire, between September 1998 and January 2000, no significant new national policy documents were published. The Labour party did publish its own version of the Patient's Charter, entitled 'The New NHS Charter' (Department of Health 1998), but the targets for waiting remained the same as those in the Conservatives' Charter.

In Porsetshire the implementation of the three part policy initiative, to tackle their waiting problem, was a staggered process. The demand management strategy that was intended to start in the September of 1998 was delayed as the steering group focused all its attention on their plans to develop a paramedic clinic. The latter arm of the overall policy initiative had been a policy proposal that was acceptable to both GPs and consultants (see Table 10.3), while the demand management proposal, though strategically desirable, had not been strongly supported by either group of clinicians (see Table 10.3). Furthermore, as time had gone on, the demand management proposal lost what little support it had received from the GPs. Communication between GPs in their professional network, which extended across the UK (see arrow (e) in Figure 10.3), revealed that in both Armagh and Kings Lynn, GPs had found that their worst fears about demand management increasing the pressures on them were confirmed. GPs reported that their attempts to rationalise the referrals they made to hospital services, through their use of demand management slots, meant that they found themselves coming under increasing pressures from patients who felt that they needed to be seen at the hospital. In the light of such evidence, Porsetshire GPs increasingly began to reject the local proposal for demand management, which to them seemed to offer a solution to the hospital's waiting list problem at their expense. Members of the steering group who represented the GP network slowly adopted a number of strategies that, intentionally or unintentionally, began to undermine the implementation of the demand management proposal. They agreed to develop the processes through which demand management slots would be administered in the community. They also agreed to work with their GP colleagues and with steering group consultants to develop referral guidelines for use with demand management slots. Over the 12–14 months that followed, they made less and less progress with these tasks until work ground to a halt. The consultants, who saw no real advantage to themselves in the demand management proposal, did little to ensure its implementation. The mangers involvement in demand management implementation was adversely affected by a change in personnel. The LHA manager, who had originally convened the meeting between managers, GPs and consultants, retired due to ill health. Her successor was slow to appreciate the network concerns that had moulded the policy proposals developed within the steering group and was slow to recognise that the demand management proposal was in danger of stalling.

As can be seen from Table 10.3, the paramedic clinic proposal was less contentious for the steering group and so was implemented with far less difficulty than the demand management proposal. The GP network actively supported it. Most of the GPs who were interviewed, saw it as a structure through which they could gain guidance in the management of patients with complex problems, but who were not suitable for surgery. All the consultants who were interviewed saw the clinic as a positive gain in hospital resources. They all saw it as a way of relieving their outpatient waiting list from the burden of patients referred to the orthopaedic department, who did not require surgery. Many also identified it as a useful route for providing some form of alternative treatment for complex patients, who had been seen in outpatients but who did not require surgery. For the managers informally interviewed, it represented an innovation which both GPs and consultants were willing to support. For the newly appointed LHA manager it was a viable proposal, which was uncontroversial, and one with which she could quickly engage and make tangible progress. In the light of these factors it is perhaps unsurprising that paramedic staffs were quickly appointed and that the clinic was up and running by January 1999, only three months after the steering group had agreed to adopt the proposal.

The appointment of the ninth consultant was also relatively uncontested (see Table 10.3) and straightforward to implement; although it took some time to construct the funding bid and to secure the finance for the post. The new consultant was eventually appointed in the spring of 2000. Interestingly at this point in time, and indeed by the spring of 2002 when the researcher departed the Porsetshire policy arena, the demand management component of the policy initiative had still not been implemented.

Conclusion

This case study clearly identifies what a politically and clinically sensitive subject waiting is. It is therefore perhaps unsurprising to see how complex it is to formulate and implement solutions, which are acceptable to the key stakeholders and interested networks. The extent to which policy-makers need to collaborate, setting aside personal and professional agendas, is clearly illuminated by this case. However, it has only been through the use of policy network theory and the use of qualitative approaches to data collection and analysis, that the complexity of factors influencing policy formulation and implementation has been appreciated.

Through this case study, the way in which both national and local structures influence policy processes and policy outcomes has been recognised. This case study has also revealed how interactions between policy networks (and the individuals within those networks), can inform policy processes and policy outcomes. Moreover, the study of the concerns and ideas circulating within networks has proved useful in gaining an understanding of the compromises and decisions that are made by policy-makers during policy formulation and implementation.

Finally, although policy network theory has more usually been used to examine national policy-making, this case study has illustrated that it can be useful in examining local actors' interpretation of national policy, and their reformulation and implementation of it, to suit local requirements. The use of Rhodes' typology in this case has proved useful in identifying that structures that are comparable to those in the national arena, exist in the local policy arena. However, further research is desirable to explore this matter further.

References

Baker, M. (2000), 'Making Sense of the NHS White Papers', *Radcliffe Medical Press Ltd*, Oxford.

Bourn, J. (2001), 'Inpatient and Outpatient Waiting in the NHS: Report by the Comptroller and Auditor General', The National Audit Office, London.

Bradshaw, P.L. and Bradshaw, G. (2004), *Health Policy for Health Care Professionals*, SAGE Publications Ltd, London.

Charmaz, K. (2000), 'Grounded Theory: Objectivist and Constructivist Methods', in Lincoln, Y. and Guba E. (eds) *Handbook of Qualitative Research*, Sage: Thousand Oaks, California.

Department of Health (1998), 'Press Release: Report on New Charter for the NHS Launched', Department of Health.

Greenaway, J., Smith, S. and Street, J. (1992), *Deciding Factors in British Politics: A Case Study Approach*, Routledge, London.

Hay, C. (2002), *Political Analysis: A Critical Introduction*, Palgrave, Hampshire.

John, P. (1998), *Analysing Public Policy*, Continuum, London.

Klein, R., Day, P., Redmayne, S. (1996), *Managing Scarcity: Priority Setting and Rationing in the National Health Service*, Open University Press, Buckingham.

Langan, M. (2001), *Welfare: Needs, Rights and Risks*, Routledge, London.

Marsh, D. (1998), 'The Development of Policy Network Approach', in Marsh, D (ed.) *Comparing Policy Networks*, Open University Press, Buckingham, 3–21.

Marsh, D. and Smith, M.J. (2000), Understanding Policy Networks: Towards a Dialectical Approach, *Political Studies*, **48**, 4–21.

Mason, J. (2002), *Qualitative Researching*, Sage Publications Ltd, London.

Rhodes, R. and Marsh, D. (1992), 'Policy Networks in British Politics: A Critique of Existing Approaches', in Marsh, D. and Rhodes, R. (eds) *Policy Networks in British Government*, Clarendon Press, Oxford, 1–26.

Rhodes, RAW. (1997), *Understanding Governance: Policy Networks, Governance, Reflexivity and Accountability*, Open University Press, Maidenhead, Berkshire.

Secretary of State for Health (1997), *The New NHS. Modern. Dependable*, Stationery Office, London.

Secretary of State for Health (1998), *A First Class Service*, Stationery Office, London.

Strauss, A.L. and Corbin, J. (1998), *Basics of Qualitative Research: Techniques and Procedures for Developing Grounded Theory*, Sage: Thousand Oaks, California.

Chapter 11

Sleepwalking to Diversity?

Gillian Olumide

Turning and turning in the widening gyre
The falcon cannot hear the falconer;
Things fall apart; the centre cannot hold.[1]

A pe ko to jeun, ki je ibaje[2]

Things fall apart as the poet suggests, the author hints at and the proverbial wisdom seeks to shed light upon. The somewhat apocalyptic imagery above seems in keeping with recently proposed shifts in thinking about the nature of difference and the recently perceived need, within Government, to try and prevent society from falling apart. Things have changed. Indeed they have. And so strange are the political times we live in that little seems to stand in the way of contrary and contradictory approaches to the maintenance of social difference.

My subject is 'diversity' and its paradoxical construction in UK policy and politics. As this is a book devoted mainly to the politics of health services, we will use the NHS as an example of an organisation advocating diversity at the behest of a government that currently regards too much diversity as damaging to 'social capital', incisively defined by a senior (ex) minister as 'the glue which holds society together'.[3] This in itself raises interesting questions as to the nature of society and the extent to which it is 'held together' or is in a state of perpetual conflict and turmoil. Whilst we may crave social order, we face the chaos and anxiety of wishing for improvement and change in our socially ascribed positions and of emphasising our group membership from a range of alternative affinity or ethnic groups. A key political question apparently gathers around how to fine tune diversity so that we have just enough of it and so that it is properly organised and regulated. To assist in this process there is a raft of new legislation. And there has always been recourse to the law in the interests of managing diversity (see Olumide, 2002, Chapter 4 for a discussion of this).

---

1 W.B. Yeats, 'The Second Coming', in A. Norman Jeffries (ed.) (1974), *W.B. Yeats: Selected Poetry*, Pan Books, London.

2 Yoruba proverb. Literally, 'the person who eats late will not eat spoiled food' or, perhaps more accessibly in this context, 'it is better to be patient and seek a lasting solution to problems rather than to cobble together a solution based on insufficient evidence and depth of thought'.

3 David Blunkett in a speech to IPPR on 7 July 2004. Home Office Publication 2004 *New Challenges for Race Equality and Community Cohesion in the Twenty-first Century.*

Diversity is not a self evident (if rather fuzzily defined) 'good', and nor are we likely to find either strength or destruction in the fact that humans have different capacities and attributes. Perceived social difference organises social inequality and this has long been the case, as Rousseau identified in 1754:

> I conceive that there are two kinds of inequality among the human species; one, which I call natural or physical, because it is established by nature, and consists in a difference of age, health, bodily strength, and the qualities of the mind or of the soul: and another, which may be called moral or political inequality, because it depends on a kind of convention, and is established, or at least authorised by the consent of men. This latter consists of the different privileges, which some men enjoy to the prejudice of others; such as that of being more rich, more honoured, more powerful or even in a position to exact obedience.

What needs to be unravelled from Rousseau's exposition, given that diversity policies were not his primary focus, is the extent to which the 'natural inequalities' produce differences in privilege and wealth. Judging by the targets of UK legislation, it is differences in age, perceived race, gender, sexuality, belief, perceived ability and mental health status which attract discrimination and inequality of life chances and which must be addressed. In effect, people enjoying the benefits of the second kind of inequality are in a position to make policies and laws to improve the position of the first groups. Whilst there is some cross-over between the two kinds, people in the first category are often excluded from the second. And what a long time policy and the law have taken to achieve their versions of equality in seeking to address this.

Rousseau edges us on the one hand to study the essentialisation of some perceived differences and the social construction of a weight of expectations on the backs of those 'natural' differences. On the other hand we must also be mindful of the 'kind of convention' which privileges some over others. What 'kind of convention' enables some differences to produce prosperity and good standing whilst others pre dispose towards poverty and lack of opportunity? Contrary to the Blunkettian view of social life, the differently perceived tend to value justice and recognition over cohesion, and hence the disability rights, feminist, anti racist, anti age discrimination and many other lobbies, including the trades union movement in its heyday, dispute their ascribed positions in the order of things and seek different settlements. They wish to bring about social change.

Cooper (2004) in addressing the underlying inequalities implied in the term 'diversity' (the usual suspects of race, gender, class and, for Cooper, sexual orientation) suggests that for diversity to become possible, these inequalities must be done away with. Suggesting, as she does, that social difference is socially constructed, Cooper effectively suggests that difference might be un-constructed or deconstructed in the interests of establishing equality of power as well as distributive equality and equality of opportunity and of recognition. This question of analysing the conditions of emergence of inequality and maldistribution of power seems particularly overlooked in the area of social policy and the poor linkage between research evidence and policy is not, by any means, a new observation.

The question of diversity, then, is complex and involves an investigation of the shift from the old order of equal opportunities and multiculturalism to managing diversity and on to the subsequent assertion that 'too much diversity' weakens the social framework. Further, how this new rhetoric of difference has impacted on organisations, including the NHS. If too much diversity is bad for society, is it also bad for organisations and workplaces?

The Sense of Diversity

Part of the conundrum of diversity is that its meanings shift. In particular, they shift in organisational and political rhetoric. This makes the use of the term problematic and unstable, as noted in the question ending the last section it is rather difficult to know what is meant by the term in different contexts. A sample of statements originating in NHS documents gives some sense of the ambiguity surrounding the diversity construct. From the NHS Employers website:[4]

> Equality and diversity are at the heart of the NHS strategy. Investing in the NHS workforce allows us to deliver a better service and improve patient care in the NHS […].
>
> Equality is about creating a fairer society in which everyone has the opportunity to fulfill their potential. Diversity is about recognising and valuing difference in its broadest sense.

The coupling of equality and diversity in NHS documents is not, incidentally, universal amongst organisations. In a report from the Department of Health Human Resources Directorate (2003) this linked position is made plain:

> Equality is about creating a fairer society where everyone can participate and has the opportunity to fulfill their potential. It is backed by legislation designed to address unfair discrimination based on membership of a particular group.
>
> Diversity is about the recognition and valuing of difference in its broadest sense. It is about creating a working culture and practices that recognize, respect, value and harness difference for the benefit of the organization and the individual, including patients.
>
> Equality and Diversity are not interchangeable-they need to be progressed together. There is no equality of opportunity if difference is not recognized and valued.

It becomes important, in this climate – where equality of opportunity is contingent upon recognizing and dealing respectfully with difference – to enquire what it is that some people are considered to be different *from* (and presumably others are not different from, or are we all just different?) Is this recognition the best way of achieving the level field of equal opportunity or the equitable distribution of resources such as pay and educational opportunities or Cooper's equality of power? There are several aspects of these fragments of text which require some scrutiny. For economy I will content myself with drawing attention to two: the repeated reference to diversity 'in its broadest sense' and the absence of any recognition of the need to name and analyse whiteness as a form of difference. The former may refer to

4 This excerpt may be viewed at http://nhsemployers.org/excellence/equality-diversity.cfm.

Rousseau's 'natural differences', surely it cannot mean diversity in all its possible manifestations? The latter, were it to be the subject of enquiry in social and health policy, might lead to the view that there is no equality of differences but rather that some differences tend to prove of greater weight and worth than others. Whiteness is the elephant in the diversity room.

Can this recognition of difference be confined to a workplace, or do the life circumstances of the differently perceived intrude? It is this latter question that links the preoccupation with too much diversity outside the workplace to the matter of not-yet-enough diversity at work. Even in the work place, the reference to 'diversity in its broadest sense' throws up the question of just how different one may be before organisational discomfort sets in: there are points at which one person's diversity upsets another's freedom. Those who smoke, swear, express certain political or religious views or wear clothing considered inappropriate in some way (the hijab for example and, within living memory, turbans, dreadlocks and women wearing trousers) may find their mode of expression curtailed or criticised. Diversity has its tacit norms of acceptable behaviour and conventions defining its limits. There is an overarching presumption of normality and 'the limits of decency' and just how different one can be which needs to be unearthed. If we are to be allowed to express and be valued for our differences, we need also to know both how our sameness or commonality with everyone else is perceived and emphasised and the criteria in use for discerning and limiting excessive difference.

Those who are considered different at work, and whose unique perspectives are now to be respected and valued in the workplace, may also be considered to be different outside work. It may be the case that the disadvantages which occur (or may have once occurred) in the workplace are simply replicated from the world at large. In which case, in order to dismantle these social disadvantages, an evidence-based approach might be of value, particularly in an industry that holds evidence in very high regard.

From Thurrock Council (not chosen for its particularly unique character nor its representativeness) the approach to diversity is somewhat reversed. It is explicitly out of socially located differences that diversity arrives in the work place[5]:

> *What is diversity?*
>
> Diversity results from differences in gender, ethnic or national origin, religion, age, disability, marital status, sexuality and many other factors which cause people to have different perspectives on the same set of facts or issues.
>
> *What does it mean to 'value diversity'*
>
> Valuing diversity means valuing the qualities that different people bring to their jobs, to the resolution of problems and to the development of business opportunities – rather than judging people and ideas by the extent to which they conform to existing values or personal preferences. It can also mean valuing differences between people and the ways

5 http://thurrock.gov.uk/i-know/diversity/content.php?page=faq. This is a section of the Thurrock diversity pages devoted to frequently asked questions.

> in which those differences can contribute to a richer, more creative and more productive business environment, which is closer to our many different customers in Thurrock.
>
> *What does 'managing diversity' mean?*
>
> The basic concept of managing diversity accepts that the workforce consists of a diverse population of people. The diversity consists of visible and non-visible differences which include, gender, ethnicity, disability, sexuality, age and religion. It is founded on the principle that harnessing these differences will create a more productive environment in which everybody feels valued, where their talents are being fully utilised, and in which organisational goals are met.

These organisational statements seem to suggest that 'natural differences' produce distinctive perspectives deriving from social circumstances. If properly managed, they may be turned to good effect and enhance the business purpose of the organisation. Diversity management, then, is not the altruistic rhetorical position of equal opportunities, but a means of meeting customer requirement and advancing organisational aims. In this understanding, diversity management may be interpreted as a means of exploiting (or 'harnessing') the differences that arise from social inequalities.

Another aspect worth considering in the two realms of diversity (inside and outside organisational settings) is that people do not arrive in an organisation by chance. The circumstances of their birth will already have contributed to the shaping of their education, economic resources, geographical location, and social experiences more generally. As employees they are selected to meet organisational criteria for the job and this includes educational attainment, prior experience and demeanour. They have already been socially sifted and have made their own assessments of realistic aspirations. As users of services supplied by the organisation, similar background influences will part determine both the experience of services and even the need for services. Most certainly these background differences will also position the user in relation to the organisation. Outside this funnelled positioning of people inside and in relation to organisations, the chaos of uncontrolled diversity poses threats and challenges that are not so easily managed. Nor, however valuable perceived differences are now to be regarded, do those differences attract equal status.

The subject demands an analysis not simply of how diversity may be promoted (surely it already exists) but of why different perceived differences have led to such striking and persistent inequalities in the first place (and why other differences are scarcely remarked upon). It may be of value to look to history, and in particular to development and re-emergence of ideologies underpinning differences. Of particular personal interest is the career of the ideology of race, and it is this strand of diversity which is often used interchangeably with the term diversity itself. It is race that forms the subject of political concerns about the poor cohesive qualities of diverse populations. Race, in turn, is often covered by reference to 'culture' or ethnicity, each of which may become imbued with racial meanings. As Gilroy (1987) has suggested about the need for historical perspectives:

> Race has to be socially and politically constructed and elaborate work is done to secure and maintain the different forms of racialisation which have characterised capitalist development. Recognising this makes it all the more important to compare and evaluate the different historical situations in which race has become politically pertinent (p. 38).

Race, and the racialisation of human difference, has always been a corrosive ideology constructed without an evidence base and justifying some of the worst crimes against humanity. There is no need to rehearse the more apparent manifestations of this, such as the Nazi implemented holocaust of world war two or the elaborate justifications for engaging in transatlantic slavery, or even the myriad day to day uses to which racial ideology is put. At present race is politically pertinent at several sites including the older (although frequently revamped) discourses around migration and the seeking of asylum (Cheong et al., 2007) and the newer rhetoric of cohesion and integration as well as a discursive 'war on terror'. It may be that the management of diversity is a further and complimentary opportunity to construct and underline racialised (and other) differences in the work place; certainly the rhetoric of diversity prepares the ground for the reification of perceived social differences and enables the regulation of difference. The possibility of a lasting solution seems to reside not with the encouragement of a toleration of diversity but with a clearer comprehension of the grounds for *in*tolerance.

Within the health services, race is evident in areas such as the under representation of black and minority ethnic people in professional and managerial posts (Oikelome, 2007), in the movement of junior doctors to more senior medical posts (Coker, 2001), in the experiences of black (particularly) male users of mental health services,[6] the experiences of minority ethnic staff of racism (Tacking Racial Harrasment in the NHS, 2001), in minority communities accessing health information (National Cancer Alliance, 2001), in experiencing inequalities in health (Postnote number 276), in the discourse around internationally recruited nurses (Pike & Ball, 2007) and so on. No matter that people from the Caribbean and the Indian sub continent were expressly recruited to staff the NHS in its early days, their progression through the ranks of health service employment has not met reasonable expectations after more than 50 years. Difference has been managed to the detriment of some groups and to the benefit of others.

Before Diversity

Whilst there may well be a sound business case for managing diversity efficiently, the rhetoric of diversity does not address social fault lines, and nor does it purport to do so (leaving the updated anti discrimination legislation, translated into organisational policies to cover this area). Diversity walks hand in glove with the denigration of multiculturalism in political circles. Like its rhetorical sister, multiculturalism is a volatile and unstable construct.

---

6 Independent Inquiry into the Death of Rodney Bennett, 2003, Cambridge, Norfolk, Suffolk and Cambridgeshire Strategic Health Authority.

Claims and counter-claims around multiculturalism have been hammered out elsewhere (for example in Barry, 2001; Kelly, (ed.) 2002; Parekh, 2000; Kymlicka, 1995 and by many, many others) and depend substantially on the philosophical traditions of the discussants and the interpretation of the term in use. For our purposes, Sivanandan (2006) critically and succinctly documents the progression of multiculturalism. He notes that this was practised in the 1960s by newly migrant Caribbeans , Asians and sympathetic whites *joining forces* to oppose racial discrimination. This 'street' response was taken into schools where respect and information about cultural difference was emphasised. A victim of its own success, this version became institutionalised, and a bottom-up movement for change became sets of top-down government policy with, as Sivanandan suggests, the political, anti racist content tamed to leave an (over) emphasis on cultural difference and distinct ethnic communities competing for funding. This, the article argues, was a shift from multiculturalism to an official culturalism, a somewhat inflexible notion of ethnicity and cultural difference.

Clearly, as the 'riots' of 2001, and 7/7 London tube bombs seem to indicate, official multiculturalism was not an unqualified success in all corners of UK. Whilst official versions of multiculturalism succeeded in transforming political will into a squabbling ethnic separatism, responsibility for the outcomes of this policy strand has been handed to the communities themselves for failing to 'integrate'. The Cantle Report (2001), Trevor Philips 'sleepwalking to segregation' speech,[7] a series of Home Office publications[8] and the day to day political rhetoric of senior government representatives have pulled the agenda away from extolling the 'vibrancy' of multicultural Britain to lamenting the inward looking self segregation of selected ethnic groups and ways in which this damages the elusive 'social cohesion'. Integration, citizenship and respect for British Values are the new assimilationist agenda. 'They' must become more like 'us'.

Werbner (2005) cites the work of Frankenberg detailing aspects of life in a Welsh border community to suggest the bounded yet flexible nature of communities. This is compared, in the paper, with Werbner's own work with the changing dynamics of Pakistani communities in South Manchester. Perhaps the differences between the two are insufficiently emphasised since Frankenberg's Welsh community unlike Werbner's Pakistani migrant community is unlikely to have been racialised and accused of failing to integrate. 'Traditional' white communities are rarely constructed as threatening to the social order or destructive of social cohesion. Their lack of 'integration' is unremarked upon, indeed the whole notion of integration begins to appear increasingly flimsy in the light of the rich tradition of community studies

---

7 22 September 2005. Manchester Town Hall. Trevor Philips, then chairperson of the Commission for Racial Equality, delivered a speech entitled 'After 7/7: Sleepwalking to Segregation'.

8 Home Office Cm 5387, 2001, *Secure Borders, Safe Haven: Integration With Diversity in Modern Britain*, London Home Office.

Home Office 2004, *Strength in Diversity: Towards a Community Cohesion and Race Equality Strategy*, London, Home Office.

Home Office Findings 253, 2005, *Diversity, trust and community participation in England*, London, Home Office.

showing the very different perceptions of local social organisation available within the UK alone. It is important to note, as much for diversity management in the work place as for the attempt to control social diversity, that an emphasis on difference problematises and fixes, or makes awkward, the perceived difference. It is also important to note that the use of the term 'community' is also unstable and shifting. When applied to a Welsh geographical location it is innocuous; when applied to groups who are portrayed as refusing to 'integrate' it is less so. Community has also become grist to the mill of racialisation.

At this point we may have stumbled across the essence of diversity both inside and outside organisations. Differences, natural differences, are the stuff of ideology. Ideological constructions of difference may bear scant resemblance to those who are differently perceived but they serve to reduce uncertainty and perhaps to structure social responses. Sivanandan (2006 op. cit.) observes the following, in the context of discussing the slide from multiculturalism to official 'culturalism' in policy.

> In 1980, in the IRR's journal *Race and Class,* we wrote that 'just to learn about other peoples' cultures is not to learn about the racism of one's own. To learn about one's own culture on the other hand, is to approach other cultures objectively.

It is just this kind of awareness which seems to be lacking in the move towards inserting statements about the management of diversity within NHS (and other organisations') policy statements. Rather than being 'understood' or 'valued', it appears to be of far greater benefit to those with different needs, attributes and other qualities defined in terms of difference, to have structural constraints and prejudices analysed and then remedied. Then the allegations of 'political correctness gone mad' will give way to a more lasting discussion of how to address fairness and equity. The 'Winterval debacle' could never have seen the light of day with a deeper and more intelligent understanding of how people might live and work together. That episode was more an example of 'official inflexibility around cultural difference gone mad.'

Apocalypse Now: Cohesion and too Much Diversity

Ideas are important, and the origins and sources of ideas which come to be of enormous influence in human affairs deserve our attention as users, workers and students of health matters and of life more generally. A key plank in the diversity paradox stems from the work on social capital by Robert Putnam, an academic from the United States who has studied the decline of community life. Like Gidden's Third Way before it, Putnam's social capital thesis has been embraced for its explanatory potential in politics. Whilst a rhetoric of diversity was becoming embedded in organisational thinking, a new panic over a lack of social capital (this is Blunkett's 'glue' referred to earlier) has emerged. The blame for this resides not with small communities in Scotland or Wales living distinctive lives but with migrants, asylum seeking groups and what might be termed 'communities of colour'. A strange and jagged line has been drawn between 'British Norms and Values' (and the toleration of difference and love of fair play are interesting aspects of this putative mono-culture which is being described in citizenship literature and the tabloids – why then do we need to manage diversity?) Assimilation is the name of the game here and we have political ferment that takes us way back before the 1960s to where the expectation was that migrants would become 'assimilated' by adopting a 'British Way of Life'. Roy Jenkins, when home secretary, argued not for assimilation but for integration and this has since been viewed as the preferred option, an understanding which lasted until very recently.

In a critique of Putnam's work, Hallberg and Lund (2005) focus on his suggestion that ethno-racial diversity is damaging to community life (which, in the UK context, seems to be used to refer to an imagined homogenous national community). The authors locate Putnam's work on social capital in what they term 'the apocalyptic genre of public discourse' (p. 54) which tends to construct 'cultural emergencies' responded to with recourse to the construction of 'traditional values' (such as 'British Norms and Values'). Whilst *Bowling Alone* (Putnam, 2000) placed Putnam in a position to influence politicians, it was later research that suggested a link between ethnic diversity and the decline of community trust. About the specifics of this suggested link, Putnam has been rather coy, although leakage of his findings has been well managed.

There can be no doubt that new Labour has embraced Putnam's influence and, in the case of Mr Blunkett, has mentioned Putnam's work directly (although not with the critical edge of Hallberg and Lund). In the current politico-cultural 'emergency', and in the context of fighting a 'war on terror' (akin to Don Quixote's tilting at windmills) against those perceived as rogue islamists (mainly, it seems) the 'common sense' position is that diversity is fine, still vibrant even, as long as those wishing to live in Britain (EU citizens are exempt from the following proviso) accept that they should be prepared to integrate and undertake citizenship education to apprise them of 'How We Do Things'. At the bottom of this 'emergency' activity seems to be a suspicion that minority ethnic communities possess too much glue and represent too much diversity with not enough of the right , integrated kind. In all its diversity, this seems to be the new Labour version of playing the race card.

Are We Sleepwalking to Diversity?

What conclusions are to be drawn between the policies of diversity management within organisations and the ferment of too much diversity in the world at large? Surely the portrayal of minority ethnic groups as insular and unwilling to join with the British People must contribute to their experiences inside organisations where these same differences are to be respected and valued.

The Vital Connection does sterling work in laying forth the aims of the NHS for its staff and service users in the area of diversity, even volunteering to use its considerable clout as a force for good outside the organisation. Just how far these aims will be frustrated by the new political perception of diversity is yet unclear. The anxiety being fostered over racialised difference in the social world cannot but affect the way racialised difference is perceived at work. Whether diversity policies can act as proxy for the 'tolerance and love of fair play of the British people', is even less clear. It may now be illegal to act in a discriminatory manner, but are the law and policy able to alter attitudes and beliefs about difference, particularly where this is constructed in such ambiguous terms? In an article about 'official' views of ethnicity (the Winterval effect), as opposed to what people are able to achieve for themselves in the way of flexible and voluntary interaction, Munira Mirza (2006) makes the following observation:

> The point of the 'diversity industry' is supposed to be a more inclusive society, in which racial barriers are broken down. Yet here we are, at the beginning of the twenty-first century, stubbornly stuck in the same prism of difference and disconnection (p. 14).

A little further into this piece Mirza makes another observation which captures a point I have been trying to argue throughout, and is therefore offered as a conclusion: that we humans don't necessarily wish for our differences to be managed by well meaning others. This is particularly so where the well meaning others do not seem to appreciate the incoherent mess they are making of the whole business of diversity, and resort to ideological construction and mystification of different differences.

> Diversity policies emerge as a kind of mood music – an attitude about what people are really like and how they relate to each other. As a result, they are rarely challenged. Complaints are made *sotto voce,* about this or that particular outrage. But overall, the assumption remains firmly in place that people are so attached to their cultural identities and incapable of transcending them, that they need special help from the authorities. The political elite congratulates itself on being open-minded to new cultures but finds it hard to believe that the lower orders are capable of making the same adjustment. The instinct is therefore to introduce pre-emptve measures to quell any tensions before they might appear.Such an assumption belies the reality, which is that historically it was usually the 'lower orders' that integrated most with new ethnic groups. They lived in closer proximity in urban connurbations and cohabited the same socio-economic brackets, meaning they tended to work together, go to school together, and even mary each other (p. 16).

Might it even be that diversity policies and politics make things worse rather than better? On the broader stage, the 2006 Equality Act, following a consultation introduced by the October 2002 document *Equality and Diversity: Making it Happen*. (HMSO) has paved the way for the establishment of a new super-quango – the Commission for Equality and Human Rights. A well as combining the work of the former Commission for Racial Equality, Equal Opportunities and Disability Rights Commission and overseeing gender, race and disability 'duties', the new commission will also monitor the 1998 Human Rights Act. Like the concept of diversity, this body seems to combine the range of human differences and ensure in the interests of fair play for all. Unlike diversity policies, it is undergirded by some serious legislative weight.

This new direction for equalities, along with the other initiatives, such as citizenship education and tests for new migrants aimed towards creating an over arching Britishness, has the potential to shape the way equality is discussed. However questions such as poverty, health inequalities and discrimination on the grounds of class appear to remain outside its remit and are catered for by other schemes such as the quest to reduce child poverty. The big issues are out there. Whether the new Commission will change minds in the workplace and in society is untested. We shall see.

References

Barry, B. (2001a), *Culture and Equality*, Polity, Cambridge.

Barry, B. (2001b), 'The Muddles of Multiculturalism', *New Left Review*, **8**, March–April.

Cantle, T. (2001), *Community Cohesion: A Report of the Independent Review Team Chaired by Ted Cantle*, The Home Office.

Cheong, P., Edwards, R., Goulbourne, H. and Solomos, J. (2007), 'Immigration,social cohesion and social capital: a critical review', *Critical Social Policy*, **27**(24) 24–49.

Coker, N. (ed.) (2001), *Racism in Medicine*, Kings Fund, London.

Cooper, D. (2004), *Challenging Diversity: Rethinking Equality and the Value of Difference*, Cambridge University Press, Cambridge.

Department of Health, Human Resources Directorate (2003), *Equality and Diversity in the NHS – Progress and Priorities*, Department of Health Publications.

Frankenberg, R. (1957), *Village on the Border: A Social Study of Religion, Politics and Football in a North Wales Community*, Cohen and West.

Kelly, P. (ed.) (2002), *Multiculturalism Reconsidered*, Polity Press, Cambridge.

Olumide, J. (2002), *Raiding the Gene Pool*, Pluto Press, Sterling, London.

Parekh, B. (2000), *Rethinking Multiculturalism*, Harvard University Press, Cambridge, MA.

Gilroy, P. (1987), *There Ain't No Black in the Union Jack: The Cultural Politics of Race and Nation*, Hutchinson Education, London.

Hallberg, P. and Lund, J. (2005), 'The business of apocalypse: Robert Putnam and diversity', *Race and Class*, **46**(4) 52–67.

Oikelome, D. (2007), *The Recruitment and Retention of Black and Minority*, Department of Health (2001), *Ethnic Staff in the NHS*, Race Equality Foundation Briefing Paper (2001), Tackling Racial Harassment in the NHS: An Evaluation of Black and minority Staff Attitudes and Experiences.

National Cancer Alliance (2001), *Ethnicity and Cancer Patient Information*, NCA, London.

Pike, G. and Ball, J. (2007), *Black and Minority Ethnic and Internationally Recruited Nurses*, Royal College of Nursing, London.

Postnote no. 276, *Ethnicity and Health*, Parliamentary Office of Science and Technology, London.

Putnam, D. (2000), *Bowling Alone: the Collapse and evival of American Community*, Simon and Schuster, New York.

Rousseau, J.J. (1754), Address to the Dijon Academy: A Dissertation on the Origin and Foundation of the Inequality of Mankind, This can be accessed at http://gutenberg.com/Books/BlackMask_online/inequ.htm.

Sivanandan, A. (2006), 'Britain's Shame', *Catalyst*, Commission for Racial Equality, July–August 2006, 18–20.

Werbner, P. (April 2005), 'The translocation of culture: "community cohesion" and the force of multiculturalism in history', *The Sociological Review*, **53**, 745–769.

Chapter 12

Politics, Ethics and Evidence: Immunisation and Public Health Policy

Alison Hann and Stephen Peckham

Public health interventions are rarely without harmful as well as a beneficial effect. As Kelly and Giacomini (2005) argue 'when many people – as well as societal constructs such as institutions and economies – are affected in many ways by every decision, the moral quandaries arise not in the question of *whether* to harm or benefit but *how* to harm *and* benefit: whom, how much, how certainly, in what ways, and so forth … The quintessential ethical problem of the public policy maker is how to define, identify, justify, and distribute inevitable benefits and harms, rather than simply striving to ensure benefit and avoid harm' (p. 254). This is a well recognised dilemma in all public policy but public health raises important questions about not only the degree or distribution of harm or benefit but also how to define those harms and benefits. For example, a key debate in public health is the extent to which it is right to intervene with a person's liberty to protect them, and/or others, from harm. In addition policy makers may formulate policy that needs to *look* good not necessarily *be* good for purely self interested political goals or because seeming to do something is seen as promoting the greatest benefit.

In this chapter we examine some of these issues using vaccination programmes as a case study. It is not our intention to question the benefit, or otherwise, of any particular vaccination programme or argue that any specific programme is right or wrong but rather to use the example of vaccination to explore public health ethics and to examine the link between ethics, evidence and public health policy.

There is a huge investment in vaccination programmes in the UK and worldwide as a preventive public health measure to improve population health. However, vaccination remains a controversial issue and the subject of media and political debate such as the continuing furore around the MMR vaccine. In addition, changes in policy are difficult to justify and implement as immunisation is seen to confer population benefit and thus suggestions to change dosage and frequency or stop programmes means that it is perceived that benefit will be reduced. Similarly the introduction of new vaccines raises important ethical questions relating to how evidence is obtained and clinical and population safety verified.

Governments and public health professionals continue to justify the programmes as being both medically and ethically good as the evidence supporting population vaccination is strong and with benefits far outweighing any potential harm. Policy is based on the need to maintain 'herd immunity' to confer population benefit. Put very simply, herd immunity is the notion that: 'If enough people in the community are immunised, the infection can no longer be spread from person to person and the disease dies out altogether' (WHO, 2005). Thus vaccination represents a classic case of a social dilemma: a potential conflict of interests between the private gains of individuals and the collective gains of a society. In this country, the choice to vaccinate is based on an individuals' free choice (though this is heavily influenced by orthodox medical evidence and social norms, see below), and it is important to note at this point that the individuals' choice is based on imperfect information, and the vaccination choice involves a positive externality.[1] However, people make choices based on their calculation of *individual* gains (and costs) without taking into consideration the social impact of their decisions. People choosing not to vaccinate are seen as being beneficiaries (or a kind of free rider)[2] of herd immunity, and are subjected to social disapproval. Those parents who choose not to vaccinate their children (for example) are vilified in the press or are accused by health professionals of putting their and other children at risk (Jansen et al., 2003). Questions of autonomy and parental choice and control have been tested in court where divorced parents have disagreed about the immunisation of their child. In one case the judge ruled against the wishes of both the mother and the child (who at the time was aged 10), claiming that the mother had a 'unreasoning and rigid approach' and that he could therefore 'discount her concerns' over the safety of the combined MMR vaccine (*The Guardian*, 2001). To maintain high immunisation rates and 'herd immunity' the government and health services actively promote vaccination and while voluntary in the UK, employ routine procedures and standardisation of vaccination programmes, including patient recall systems (GP targets) publicity campaigns and school based delivery programmes to ensure maximum coverage – sometimes in the face of growing evidence questioning the efficacy of programmes. For example, up until last year the BCG vaccination programme was actively promoted in secondary schools despite questions about the efficacy of the programme, which had been questioned for a number of years – finally leading to its withdrawal. Does this make the policy to promote BCG vaccination in the first place a bad policy? This returns us to the dilemma mentioned earlier. Given that the social benefit of vaccination programmes rests on herd immunity, and that this can only be achieved if a high percentage of the population at risk gets the vaccine. Should this choice be left to the individual? This begs the question – to what extent should the state coerce citizens into being

1 Immunisations give external benefits. When you get a vaccine for a certain disease, you make it less likely that you will contract the disease (internal benefit), but you also make it less likely that other people will contract the disease, because they will not catch it from you (external benefit) Most vaccines are not 100 per cent effective, that is, they do not reduce the probability of contracting the disease, if exposed, to 0, but if a high percentage of the population gets the vaccine, a disease can be eradicated because those few people who have the disease may not happen to come into contact with an unvaccinated person.

2 An individual in this case benefits from the immunisations that other people get, because their actions reduce the risk of contacting someone with the disease. The free rider saves him/herself the risk of being immunised, but still reaps the benefits of the public health measure.

vaccinated – especially if this coercion is based on imperfect information?[3] This raises important ethical questions.

The Ethical Dimension

What do we mean by ethical? Typically, a moral or ethical statement asserts that some particular action is right or wrong, or that certain kinds of action are right or wrong, or it may propose some kind of general principle from which we might determine which actions are right and which are wrong – for example we might have the principle that we must always try to aim for the greatest general happiness, or try to minimise the total suffering of all human beings (sometimes expressed as 'all those concerned') – or perhaps we should devote ourselves completely to the service and worship of God, or we must try to do what is dutiful and fulfil our obligations to others – or perhaps, it's a case of every man (sic) for himself. Now, which ever approach might be taken, it would seem self evident that any public health measure that conferred only good outcomes (such as clean drinking water) must be 'ethical' (provided that in doing so, no one was harmed or had their rights violated). Sadly, few public health measures are so cut and dried. In the case of vaccination programmes, it is known that certain vaccinations may damage or cause harm to some individuals and while most of these harmful effects are considered minor, some effects of vaccination lead to more serious complications. For example, the data sheet produced by the manufacturer for M-M-R 11 (Merck Sharpe & Dohme) lists under 'Adverse Effects' symptoms which range from 'Burning and/or stinging of short duration at the injection site' (p. 6) to 'convulsions' and 'death' (p. 6). Thus the calculation of whether a vaccination programme is 'good' or not involves some kind of balance between the benefits and harms. This is further complicated by sometimes conflicting medical evidence, individual freedom of choice, societal benefits, and the right of the state to enforce compliance, and to what degree.

One argument for population immunisation is based on the utilitarian premise that an action is right if and only if it promotes the best consequences for the largest number of people. This approach, so eloquently summarised by Spock in 'Star Trek – the movie' as '... the needs of the many outweigh the needs of the few'. This provides a specification of right action, making the link between 'rightness' and best consequences, but this, in itself doesn't give any real guidance on what counts as a 'best consequence'. Thus a second premise is required in that the best consequences are those in which happiness (or utility) is maximised. So we might modify Spocks formulation to : 'the happiness (utility) of the many outweigh the happiness (utility) of the few'.[4]

---

3 This imperfect information can apply to both the individual and the policy maker. Controversies over medical evidence may be ignored, glossed over or even suppressed.

4 Another common formulation of this is 'the greatest happiness for the greatest number', but these are all actually misleading. As Kymlicka observes this contains two distinct maximands – 'greatest happiness' and 'greatest number'. It is impossible for any theory to contain a double maximand, and any attempt to implement it quickly leads to an impasse. See Griffin (1986: 151–4).

Utilitarianism has a long and illustrious pedigree having gone through numerous permutations in the hands of philosophers, economists and politicians who have been attracted to its potential for social reform (Oliver, 2006). Its roots can be found in trying to understand human behaviour and Aristotalian ideas about human flourishing, (or eudaimonia), but has since evolved into terms such as preference satisfaction, or utility (Mill, 1974). Thus, where an agent has a choice between courses of action (or inaction) the right act is the one that will produce the most 'utility', usually understood as benefit or happiness. To achieve this, it is necessary to be able to add up all the amounts of utility it produces for all who are in 'any way affected' and similarly to add up and measure all the amounts of pain (harm/misery) the action produces, and then subtract the amount of pain from the amount of harm. The right action will then be the one for which there is the greatest positive (or the least negative) balance. This has several obvious attractions. It would seem reasonable that morality, if it is going to guide conduct, should have something to do with happiness, flourishing or benefit. It would also seem natural to seek to avoid pain or harm, and also to balance the one against the other. In taking the *general* happiness or benefit as a standard of right action, utilitarianism seems to satisfy the presumption that moral actions should be unselfish and fair (Mackie, 1977). This balancing of benefits and harm would seem ideally suited, at first consideration to public health interventions, vaccination, being an eminently suitable case in point. Balance, the misery and death caused by, say, smallpox or polio against the relatively small risks and side effects of the vaccination, and it would seem that vaccinating for smallpox must be a right action as defined above. However, what about vaccination for rarer diseases or those creating less complications such as chicken pox, flu or hepatitis B? However, before we deal with the specific problems raised by particular public health interventions, we need to consider some of the standard problems raised by utilitarianism, or its specific interpretation here of act utilitarianism (Mackie, 1977).

The difficulties are both well known and well rehearsed elsewhere, so we will mention them only briefly here. Firstly, what are we to include in 'all who are in any way affected'? Does this mean all human beings or all sentient beings? Does it include those who are now alive, or also future generations? Is it really possible to measure harm and benefit in the way required by act utilitarianism? For example, supposing vaccination benefited 20 per cent of the people hugely, and was only mildly unpleasant for 55 per cent, while 15 per cent were caused long term and severe suffering. A classic utilitarian might well judge that this was a good trade off but how we identify benefit and harm and the degree of benefit or harm are also clearly important in making such an assessment. Further difficulties are also raised by the recognition that act utilitarianism focuses primarily on the outcome and not the means to achieve it. Thus it would be possible to tolerate the use of torture or violence, if this leads to the maximisation of the general good. Thus utilitarianism not only allows, but enjoins, in some circumstances, that the benefit (utility) of 'the many' might be 'purchased' at the cost of the undeserved and uncompensated misery of 'the few'. This raises questions of rights and justice which Mill himself recognised and which have been extensively discussed in the literature (Mackie, 1977; Kymlicka, 1990).

There is also a difficulty when it comes to weighing the distribution of harm and utility within the life of any individual. A period of misery followed by one of happiness seems preferable to a period of happiness followed by one of misery, even if the *quantities* are equal. In addition are we talking about *expected* utility or *actual* utility? Clearly we do not always have perfect information concerning all the possible outcomes of actions. And lastly – there is no specification in utilitarianism that certain acts are 'immoral' even if they do promote the greatest benefit. For example there is not requirement to always tell the truth, be compassionate, keep promises or to be loyal. So, for example, if the kind of utility that is being maximised is, say, freedom from worry or distress, then a lie – if it maximises this, is preferable to the truth.

One attempt at dealing with these problems is to introduce moral rules (rule utilitarianism). This holds that the rightness of an action is *not* to be tested by simply evaluating its consequences, but by considering if it falls under a certain rule. Whether the rule is to be considered an acceptable moral rule, is, however decided by considering the consequences of adopting the rule. As Kymlicka explains it: 'we should apply the test of utility to rules, and then perform whichever act is endorsed by the rules, even if another act might produce more utility. Social co-operation requires rule-following, so we should assess the consequences, not simply of acting in a particular way on this occasion, but of making it a rule that we act in that way (p. 27). However, rule utilitarianism also has a fatal flaw. Sometimes, in order to act morally we need to make exceptions to rules – especially when rules come into conflict. In order to take account of this, the rule utilitarian may wish to add in some flexibility so that it is permissible to break the rule if following it would lead to 'bad' consequences'. A rule might be that all children should be vaccinated against measles to ensure no-one contracts measles or suffers from the complications of measles. However, some children do experience side effects from vaccination so there may be grounds in some cases not to vaccinate an individual child, but ultimately policy decisions about this require a balance between outcomes for the individual and for the population as a whole. Thus decisions are based on the consequences of not vaccinating or vaccinating. Therefore, once this qualification is added it implies that the rule is not hard and fast and may be ignored – in particular it can be ignored when the *consequences* are taken into account and therefore rule utilitarianism appears to collapses back into act utilitarianism. The only way to preserve the difference between rule utilitarianism and act utilitarianism is to insist that the rules be obeyed *without exception*. In this case, even if the consequences of following the rule will produce bad consequences, the rule utilitarian must follow them regardless of the consequences – and therefore is no longer a consequentialist, and no longer a utilitarian.

When we come to apply utilitarianism to public health interventions, this becomes even more complicated. Common sense would seem to suggest that for any public health intervention to be considered ethical, the intervention must benefit the majority of 'all who are in any way effected' and harm as few as possible. On strict utilitarian grounds this could be achieved through coercion, for example by passing legislation that forces people to adopt practices against their will (e.g. mandatory vaccination), be tested or screened against their will (for example genetic testing of infants) even in the face of (perhaps quite severe) harm to some. Furthermore, it is feasible that certain medical practices could be conducted upon unwilling research 'guinea pigs' if it were believed to be in the interests of society, (or at least 'those who are in any way effected'). In public health policy then, it would seem imperative to be able to calculate and define harm and benefit. How is this to be achieved? With utilitarianism we need to be able to quantify benefits to show that we have achieved the maximum well being or good and that this outweighs any harm. The ethical and philosophical literature has amply explored these issues in relation to the moral right to restrict the actions and liberties of others in public health based on discussion of utility, consequentionalism and rights (Hare, 1984; Mackie, 1977).

However, leaving these debates to one side, one key problem with public health policy and practice is the way that benefit and harm are identified and measured. It seems obvious to say that public health policy and action should improve the overall well being of the population. But this may, as in the case vaccination, be to the detriment of some individuals well being. In order to justify vaccination programmes we therefore need to measure and compare, or balance out, these harms and benefits even though it is not always clear that all benefits and harms are known about, in other words we may not have perfect information. As Cribb argues 'Given the complex causal and constitutive links between aspects of health, welfare, and well-being … evaluations [of the effects of interventions], as well as the predictions they rest upon, have to be multidimensional' (Cribb, 2005: 66). Essentially there are four areas of balance that need to be addressed in public health:

- benefit and harm,
- future benefit/harm over present benefit/harm,
- individual or the population,
- individual freedom or responsibility to protect the rights and freedoms of others.

These raise questions of definition and measurement. The role of an ethical framework is to guide decision making to provide the correct or best balance. The extent to which any one area is seen as more important than another will need to be reflected in the way judgements are made. This next section therefore explores the role of evidence in public health and discusses some of the methodological issues that arise in the way evidence is constituted and used in policy and practice.

Evidence Based Public Health Policy and Practice

Concern about the use of research and its influence on policy practice is not new (Oliver, 2006; Weiss, 1979). However, while it is increasingly being recognised that there are valid concerns about the basis and nature of evidence based medicine little attention has been paid to the area of public health policy.

Evidence is by nature contestable. In health care and medicine the dominant concept of evidence is that encapsulated in evidence-based medicine (EBM). This approach focuses on the individual patient and evidence is '… developed through systematic and methodologically rigorous clinical research, emphasising the use of science and de-emphasising the use of intuition, unsystematic clinical experience, patient and professional values, and patho-psychologic rationale' (Dobrow et al., 2004: 207). Critics of EBM argue that the approach is too narrow and excludes other forms of clinically relevant evidence (Miles et al., 2000). Proponents of EBM have responded by developing hierarchies of evidence based on methodological rigour but these remain value bound and not, themselves, evidence based (Oxford Centre for Evidence Based Medicine, 2001; Miles et al., 2000). Despite these debates EBM has continued to expand into clinical decision making and increasingly into the health policy arena focusing attention on evidence based health policy (Black, 2001; Nutley and Davies, 2000; Dobrow et al., 2004). Yet as Black (2001) has argued: '... evidence based policy is not simply an extension of EBM: it is qualitatively different'.

Public health by its very nature is not focused on the individual but on populations and the practice of public health is a more political process than medicine as it deals with social processes and the wider population (Hunter 2003). Values are more explicit in relation to public health than medical practice, although values are an important element of any system of health care. For example, the relative priority given to health inequalities is underpinned by ideological positions about the nature of inequality itself. Also debates about the extent to which the state should intervene in individual lifestyles is not one that is open to a strict evidence based approach without recourse to some moral or ideological standpoint. However, evidence is often employed in arguments to sustain particular view points (e.g. smoking, wearing seat belts and vaccination programmes).

Traditionally public health has relied on epidemiological studies to demonstrate the need for, and the effectiveness of, interventions. These studies are designed to show that there has been an overall benefit from particular interventions. But epidemiological evidence is not always clear as demonstrated in recent debates about the effectiveness of flu vaccination programmes. In some areas the evidence on effectiveness is much clearer (e.g. small pox, polio) whereas in others questions are raised about who should be immunised (e.g. flu, TB). But all immunisation programmes cause some harm to some individuals but the effects to these individuals may not be statistically relevant in large scale epidemiological studies although individual effects may be catastrophic. Therefore, leaving aside the broader politics for the present, decisions to introduce vaccination must be based on balancing the benefit for the many over harm for the few. However, the normal ways of identifying benefit and harm are not as clear cut as say, testing a new drug, as the methodological issues of providing evidence are complex (Dobrow et al., 2004; Price et al., 2004). Dobrow et al. (2004) suggest that evidence is either philosophical-normative (independent of context) with an emphasis on the quality and criteria for evidence or practical-operational (context-based) where evidence '... is characterised by its emergent and provisional nature, being inevitably incomplete and inconclusive (209). The latter more accurately reflects the situation in public health which relies on interpretation of evidence such as the debate about flu deaths. Douglas (1986) has suggested in fact that the way we make sense of the world, the categories of classification, are all socially constituted and socially reproduced and thus all evidence is set within specific contexts (or scientific paradigms: see Khun, Popper).

We can see how these perspectives relate to vaccination policy. Evidence about vaccine benefit and harm is collected through a variety of ways. However, initially vaccines are tested for effectiveness through clinical trials to demonstrate that they are safe and provide a specific outcome that confers benefit – usually identified as an observed immune response. The approach to clinical trials is rigorously monitored. Trials are, though conducted on carefully screened patients and do not represent a 'normal' population. For example vaccines are routinely tested on adults and dosages adjusted by body mass for children. Also it is thought that as the immune system of young children is not fully developed higher dosages are required for very young children that might be given to an adult in order to achieve an immune system response (also other unknowns like the action and side effects of adjuvants). Evidence of effectiveness is also based on theoretical assumptions about how the immune system works and there is not universal agreement on this (Matzinger, 2002). Actual safety of vaccines and population benefit relies on larger epidemiological studies and the collection of data on adverse events once the vaccine is in general use, but epidemiological studies may not be sensitive enough to identify problems and reporting systems are not foolproof (Price et al., 2004; Salisbury et al., 2002; Singleton et al., 1999). In cases where disease identification is clear (e.g. polio, TB) the population effect my be easy to identify but in some areas such as flu and flu like symptoms the situation is less clear with considerable debate about the numbers of deaths from flu and the benefits of vaccination based on interpretation of data extrapolated through assumptions about attributable deaths (Doshi, 2005; Jefferson, 2006). In all immunisation programmes there will also be individual instances of harm and central to the identification of these is the adverse reaction reporting systems (the Yellow card system in the UK) in which medical practitioners voluntarily report adverse effects of all drugs including vaccines. However, the reliability of the system, while generally good, has suffered from underreporting of adverse symptoms. It is thought that less than 10 per cent are reported. Studies have shown that concerted attempts to make practitioners and patients aware of the need to report adverse events dramatically increases this figure.

As Davies (2005) and other authors demonstrate, there are a wide range of influences working on decision makers, of which formal research evidence is a small part (Oliver, 2006). One needs to recognise the context, competing interests and political processes that are involved in making policy. Research evidence is only one of a range of sources of evidence that is used by policy makers and it competes with other sources of evidence. Public health policy making as being characterised by 'bricolage' (Levi-Straus, 1966: 16–22), a process where the policy maker '… in contrast to the scientist or engineer, acquires and assembles tools and materials as he or she goes, keeping them until they might be used.' (Freeman, in press). Moreover, as Lindblom and Cohen (1979) point out, evidence from research has to compete with 'ordinary knowledge' which owes its origins to 'common sense, casual empiricism or thoughtful speculation and analysis'. In the specific case of health services, Hanney et al. (2003) argue that there is generally more resistance to the use of social science, than to the use of natural science. But, they argue, natural science is less likely to incorporate political or ideological considerations. But this assumes that scientific evidence is not itself contestable although it would be a brave politician indeed who suggested dismantling the vaccination programme – or the breast screening programme on the grounds that it was based on 'bad' evidence, because there is a strong public perception that it is a public 'good'.

The Ethical Basis for Vaccination

We are concerned in public health about the consequences of actions and the grounds upon which public health interventions can be justified. but little attention has been paid to how resultant harms and benefits are accounted for and on what grounds public health interventions can be undertaken. This suggests some recourse to a set of rules or principles that do not bind actions as in rule utilitarianism or neglect how things are achieved as in act utilitarianism.

However, before we go any further, we need to focus on the questions being asked here with regard to vaccination programmes. Firstly, is it a 'good' policy, secondly, is it based on sound medical evidence? And thirdly is it 'good' for society?

With regard to the first question, whether or not something is a good policy or not depends, as Wildavsky (1972) has observed, on 'who is doing the judging, what yardsticks they use, and on the basis of what information'. Bearing this in mind, if public health policies are judged on the basis of their perceived benefits and whether or not they have public (and political) support, then vaccination is widely considered to be a 'good' policy. If we are to be cynical, what seems to be crucial in securing both public and political support in any public health policy, is not just its substance, but how it looks (Hann, 1999a). Political judgements are more often than not based impressions about the effects and costs of the programme, especially in the case of technical areas where specialised knowledge is needed in order to understand the complexities of possible costs and benefits. Coupled with this, policies become entrenched, and the political consequences of dismantling an ineffective programme which has strong public support might be greater than leaving it in place. However, public support of health policies (such as vaccination or screening) are based on the belief that they (the public) are being correctly informed of the possible harms and benefits. However, as it has been demonstrated elsewhere, the communication of risks and benefits are sometimes manipulated for political reasons (Hann, 1999b; Skrabanek, 1994; Furedi, 1998), and the medical evidence may not be as uncontroversial as people are led to believe. This brings us to the second question mentioned above – is the programme based on sound medical evidence? As was noted above, this issue is complicated. The drive for health promotion has brought with it a kind of obsession to vaccinate. Along with the already scheduled childhood vaccinations (diphtheria, polio, whooping cough, measles, rubella, tetanus, mumps, meningitis, pneumococcus, septicaemia and flu) there are suggestions that it might be advisable to vaccinate against sexually transmitted infections, cervical cancer, herpes, chicken pox and even bird flu. While the medical epidemiological evidence for some of these may be sound – for others it is less so and the focus on vaccination may even deflect attention from the broader social causes of infection. (Herceg, A.,

Pessaris, I. and Mead, C., 1994) . Lastly, whether or not a particular health policy is good for a particular society (as a whole) is a difficult and complex question, which turns on the precise definition of a 'good' (and 'society'), and the values that underpin it. All of which leaves us with a dilemma which it seems, cannot be solved for us by utilitarianism (act or rule).

If the aim of public health policy is to reduce deaths and morbidity from disease x, the ends cannot justify the means if we want to live in a society that values individual autonomy, justice (however conceived) and informed choice. In addition, people can make genuine mistakes based on the best available information, and with the best intentions - policies come into being which are later found to be ineffective, inappropriate or counter productive. If we are to abandon utilitarianism, how are we to judge the ethical merits of any given public health policy? One possibility is the one proposed by Rosalind Hursthouse (and others) which invokes a notion of virtue. Her formulation of virtue ethics, has its roots in the Aristotelain idea of 'moral character' or 'virtue'. While it is beyond the remit of this chapter to discuss virtue ethics in detail we might, outline briefly how it might help us out of the quandary mentioned above. Firstly it is agent centred rather than act (or rule) centred. As Hursthouse puts it virtue ethics addresses … itself to the question: 'What sort of person should I be?' rather than to the question: 'What sorts of action should I do?' (p. 17). So, while the utilitarian might claim that: 'an action is right if it promotes the best consequences', virtue ethics would instead claim that: 'an action is right if it is what a virtuous agent would characteristically do in the circumstances'.[5] While Hursthouse is reluctant to provide readers with a list of virtues, in the area of medical practice, Beauchamp and Childress (1994) provide us with a possible starting point, they suggest that what Hursthouse calls virtues could just as easily be called 'principles' and these are: respectfulness, nonmalevolence, benevolence, justice or fairness, truthfulness and confidentialness (p. 67). Oakley and Cocking (2001) also lists truthfulness, and adds trustworthiness to the list of 'medical virtues' (p. 93). However this approach is not without its difficulties, and while many of the philosophical problems need not be discussed in detail here, one that we might mention is that these virtues may also be in tension with each other or conflict. General Practitioners (for example), might have to put the patient's individual need above the needs of 'the many', for example by recommending that a particular child ought not to be vaccinated because of some pre-existing condition which is contra-indicated. As Hare (1993) points out: 'Doctors in general tend to give extra weight to the interests of their own patients …'. Put into this context, the actions of the virtuous general practitioner might be in tension with the virtuous public health policy maker? However, leaving this aside for the moment, one way to apply virtue ethics in this instance is suggested by Oakley & Cocking (1999) in their book *Virtue Ethics and Professional Roles.* They suggest that:

> One of the strengths of an approach to professional roles which takes their moral status to depend on importantly on their links with key human goods is that this sort of approach fits naturally with a central feature of any occupations claim to be a profession in the first place (p. 79).

5 Readers can find a more detailed discussion of virtue ethics in Philippa Foot (1978) *Virtues and Vices*, University of California Press, Berkley; and Rosalind Hursthouse (1999) *On Virtue Ethics*, Oxford University Press, Oxford.

That is: we expect professionals – medical or political to act in a 'professional' manner, which embraces a notion of acting morally within the context of their profession. We need to be able to rely on health professionals (and policy makers) to be *virtuous in their actions* in that they don't manipulate information, drown out opposing voices and ride roughshod over peoples' rights and autonomy.

Conclusion

An ethical approach to vaccination would, therefore, be one that demonstrates:

- that the intervention does what it says its supposed to do,
- that there is good medical evidence to support it,
- that the harms, as well as the benefits caused by the intervention are honestly and correctly understood and disseminated,
- that alternative policy options are considered openly.

However, as the discussion earlier in this chapter highlights there are still questions that remain unanswered including whether some vaccines 'do what they say they do'. An example here is flu vaccine where there is some debate about both efficacy and target populations (Jefferson, 2006). In addition, quantifying harm and benefit is difficult where evidence is contradictory or of a questionable standard (Price et al., 2004).

At the same time vaccination is considered to be a social norm – it has wide social acceptability, strong political and medical support and is widely seen as beneficial. Those questioning vaccination and vaccination policy are seen as 'cranks', anti science, or at least … Public support for vaccination programmes is paramount given the need to reach a situation of herd immunity. This makes the furore over the MMR vaccination interesting. In order to ensure continued public support a move to single vaccines may have been one way to keep public confidence and high levels of immunisation rates. While supply of single vaccines was clearly an issue this is a situation where a policy shift not based on evidence of improved efficacy may have been more useful rather than relying on medical and scientific evidence showing the MMR was safe. In the case of the TB secondary school booster programme strenuous efforts to ensure all children were vaccinated continued right up to the point of abandoning the programme based on a review of the evidence in 2005 – including pressure on parents who declined to have their children vaccinated.

Vaccination programmes are undertaken within the context of competing values where evidence, individual freedom, practicality, political expediency and support and different conceptualisation of harms and benefits co-exist (Cribb, 2005; Salmon and Omer, 2006). There is also a degree of uncertainty about the nature of and the way in which vaccination actually works. What is clear here is that a rational framework for deciding what course of action to take based n best evidence does not exist. Policy makers and practitioners are more often than not operating in an area of health care that does not conform to medical scientific paradigms. The adage that public health is politics is clearly pertinent and developing an ethical framework for action must, necessarily, be set within a social context (Cribb, 2005).

References

Beauchamp, T. and Childress, J. (1994), *Principles of Biomedical Ethics, Fourth Edition*, Oxford University Press, Oxford.

Black, N. (2001), 'Evidence based policy: Proceed with care', *British Medical Journal*, **323**, 275–9.

Cribb, A. (2005), *Health and the Good Society*, Oxford University Press, Oxford.

Davies, P. (2005), 'Survey of senior Whitehall Policy Makers', Presented by Dr Davies, Deputy Director, Chief Social Researcher's Office, Prime Minister's Strategy Unit, at a Workshop on 'Conducting and Commissioning Syntheses for Managers and Policy Makers', December 2005, Montreal, Canada.

Dobrow, M., Goel, V. and Upshur, R. (2004), 'Evidence-based health policy: Context and utilisation', *Social Science and Medicine*, **58**, 207–217.

Doshi, P., (2005), Are flu death figures more PR than science?, *British Medical Journal*, **331**, 1412.

Douglas, M, (1986), *How Institutions Think*, Syracuse University Press, Syracuse.

Freeman, R. (in press), 'The work the document does: Reflections on the relationship between research and policy in public health', *Journal of Health Politics, Policy and Law.*

Furedi, F. (1998), *Culture of Fear: Risk-taking and the morality of low expectation*, Cassell, London.

Griffin, J. (1986), *Well-being: Its meaning, Measurement, and Moral Importance*, Oxford University Press, Oxford.

Guardian (13 June 2003), *Court Orders Girls To Have MMR jab.*

Hann, A. (1999a), 'Cancer Test Smeared: Preventive medicine or an expensive mistake?' in *Critical Public Health*, **9**(3) 251–256.

Hann, A. (1999b), 'Propaganda Versus Evidence Based Health Promotion: The case of breast screening', in *International Journal of Health Planning and Management.*

Hanney, S., Gonzalez-Bloch, M., Buxton, M. and Kogan, M. (2003), 'The utilisation of health research in policy-making: Concepts, examples and methods of assessement', *Health Research Policy and Systems*, **1**(2), at www.health-policy-systems.com/content/1/1/2.

Hare, R.M. (1982), *Ethical Theory and Utilitarianism*, in Sen, A. and Williams (eds), *Utilitarianism and Beyond*, Cambridge University Press, Cambridge.

Herceg, A., Pessaris, I. and Mead, C. (1994), An Outbreak of measles in a Highly immunised population: Immunisation status and vaccine efficiency, *Australian Journal of Public Health*, **18**, 249–52.

Hunter, D.J. (2003), *Public Health Policy*: Polity Press, Cambridge.

Hursthouse, R. (1999), *On Virtue Ethics*, Oxford University Press, Oxford.

Jansen, V., Stollenwerk, N., Jensesn, H., Ramsay, M. et al. (2003), Measles Outbreaks in a Population with Declining Vaccine Uptake, *Science*, **301**(804).

Jefferson, T. (2006), Influenza vaccination: Policy versus evidence, *British Medical Journal*, **333**, 912–915.

Kenny, N. and Giacomini, M. (2005), Wanted: A new ethics field for health policy analysis, *Health Care Analysis*, **13**(4) 247–260.

Lévi-Strauss, C. (1966), *The Savage Mind*, Weidenfeld and Nicholson, London.

Kymlicka, W. (1990), *Contemporary Political Philosophy: An Introduction*, Clarendon Press, Oxford.

Lindblom, C. and Cohen, D. (1979), *Usable Knowledge: Social Science and Social Problem Solving*, Yale University Press, New Haven.

Mackie, J.L. (1977), *Ethics: Inventing Right and Wrong*, Penguin, London.

Matzinger, P. (2002), The Danger Model: a renewed sense of self, *Science*, **296**, 301–305.

Merk, Sharp and Dohme (2006), Datasheet, M-M-R 11, measles mumps and rubella virus vaccine live, 015ml subcutaneous injection. DP/1-MMR-11-0206(280206).

Miles, A., Bentley, P., Polychronis, A., Grey, J; and Melchiorri, C. (2001), Recent developments in the evidence-based healthcare debate, *Journal of Evaluation in Clinical Practice*, **7**(2) 85–89.

Mill, J.S. (ed.) (1974), *On Liberty*, Penguin Classics, London.

Nutley, S. and Davies, H. (2000), 'Making a reality of evidence-based practice: Some lessons from the diffusion of innovations', *Public Money & Management*, **20**(4) 35–42.

Oakley, J. and Cocking, D. (2001), *Virtue Ethics and Professional Roles*, Cambridge University Press, Cambridge.

Oliver, T.R. (2006), The politics of public health policy, *American Review of Public Health*, **27**, 195–233.

Price, D., Jefferson, T. and Demicheli, V. (2004), Methodological issues arising from systematic reviews of the evidence of safety of vaccines, *Vaccine,* **22**, 2080–2084.

Rhodes, R. and Marsh, D. (1992), 'New directions in the study of policy networks', *European Journal of Political Research*, **21**, 181–205.

Salisbury, D.M., Beverley, P.C.L. and Miller, E. (2002), Vaccine programmes and policies, *British Medical Bulletin*, **62**, 201–211.

Salmon, D.A. and Omer, S.B. (2006), Individual freedoms versus collective responsibility: Immunization decision-making in the face of occasionally competing values, *Emerging Themes in Epidemiology*, **3**(13) (http://www.ete-online.com/content/3/1/13).

Short, S. (1997), 'Elective affinities: Research and health policy development', in Gardner, H. (ed.), *Health Policy in Australia*, Oxford University Press, Melbourne.

Singleton, J.A., Lloyd, J.C. and Mootrey, G.T., et al. (1999), An overview of the Vaccine Adverse Event Reporting System (VAERS) as a surveillance system, *Vaccine*, **17**, 2908–2917.

Skrabanek, P. (1994), *The Death of Humane Medicine and the Rise of Coercive Healthism*, Social Affairs Unit, London.

Weiss, C. (1979), 'The many meanings of research utilization', *Public Administration Review*, **39**, 426–431.

Wildavsky. A. (1972), 'The Self-Evaluating Organization', *Public Administration Review*, **32**(5) (Sep. – Oct., 1972), 509–520.

World Health Organisation (2005), Factsheet no. 288, *Immunisation Against Diseases of Public Health Importance: The Benefits of Immunisation.*

Chapter 13

Pharmaceutical Policy in the UK

Kathryn Jones

In modern healthcare systems, governments are increasingly pursuing strategies which aim to secure access to cost-efficient and effective medicines for citizens. Over the past ten years in the UK, the New Labour Government has supported the introduction of clinical guidelines and national service frameworks for a number of condition areas and population groups, and the assessment of the efficacy of new medicines and medical technologies through the National Institute of Health and Clinical Excellence (NICE). In addition it has pursued a policy of cost containment on the price it is willing to pay for medicine prescribed through the National Health Service (NHS). This chapter considers the implications of the pursuit of these strategies for the relationship between government and the pharmaceutical industry in the UK. These changes are being introduced at a time when the global pharmaceutical industry is contracting and competition for markets growing (Busfield, 2003), and governments are increasingly concerned with securing inward investment to pursue so-called knowledge-based economies (HM Treasury, 2004).

Within the health policy process, the pharmaceutical industry is widely considered to be a powerful player with close ties to government, the professions and other stakeholders such as patients groups. Increasingly, questions are being raised over the extent of these links and the influence of industry over other stakeholders (cf. Which, 2003; Herxheimer, 2003). There have also been concerns about the lack of transparency in the relationship between industry and the DH which is charged with both negotiating with industry the price the NHS pays for branded pharmaceuticals and working with industry to support its activities (Kay, 2001a, 2001b). This tension of meeting the needs of tax-payers and supporting industry has been described as the dilemma of 'trying to serve two masters' (HC, 2005: 6). This chapter explores the links between industry and the UK Government, in particular the Department of Health (DH). It draws on interviews with industry representatives and observers which explored the role of industry in the health policy process. The chapter considers a number of questions: how is government's relationship with industry structured? Whose interests are served by the process? What external pressures are brought to bear on the relationship? How much influence does industry have in the health policy process? Before this, the economic, political and regulatory context of industry is explored. The chapter then addresses the key points of contact between industry and the DH and the way in which developments in the wider environment influence this are then discussed. The chapter concludes by arguing that industry is influential in the health policy process, but it may not be the most significant player in the process. The focus here is on interactions with the DH, although issues relating to the licensing of medicines through the Medicines and Healthcare Products Regulatory Agency (MHRA), are beyond the scope of this chapter.

The chapter draws on ten interviews undertaken in the summer of 2005 and 2006 with key individuals from the pharmaceutical sector – representatives of individual companies as well as the industry's trade association, the Association of the British Pharmaceutical Industry (n=4), government (n=3), industry observers (n=2) and an informant from the heath consumer group sector (n=1). The interviews covered a range of issues around points of contact, the role of other healthcare stakeholders and perceptions of influence. Respondents were assured of their anonymity, in the chapter, quotes from interviewees in the pharmaceutical industry are denoted by 'PI' and those from government and other stakeholders by 'PS'. The interviews lasted between 45 minutes and an hour and were taped and transcribed. An initial coding framework was developed to categorise the data according to themes emerging from the interviews.

The Economic, Political and Regulatory Context

As an actor in a globalised industry which governments rely on to drive health improvements, the pharmaceutical sector has the power to exert influence culturally, economically and politically (O'Donovan and Glavanis-Grantham, 2005). Within industrialised economies the pharmaceutical industry is a leader of innovation, manufacturing, and marketing, creating well-known brands which then permeate health systems (Moran, 1999). In addition, the industry contributes significantly to individual economies, providing employment, investing in infrastructure and research and development (R&D). For example, in 2006 the pharmaceutical sector generated a UK trade surplus of over £3 billion and spent a similar amount on R&D, around a quarter of all UK manufacturing industry expenditure on R&D (DH, 2007). Culturally the pharmaceutical sector is also a major force, providing science-based solutions to illnesses which are principally defined and understood within the dominant paradigm of the medical model. As an industry its products have contributed to health gains and improved health outcomes. However, it is also able to influence debate about the nature of ill-health, some critics warn of 'disease mongering' to build markets for products (Moynihan et al., 2002).

Within the UK, as a policy actor, the pharmaceutical industry can be considered to be a insider group (Grant, 1989). It has close and long-standing links with ministers and Whitehall, and there has long been a 'revolving-door' of officials moving between the public and private sector (Pollock, 2004). Industry is represented in many consultations by the Association of the British Pharmaceutical Industry (ABPI), which has a membership of over 100 companies operating in the UK. Given the revenue advantages of industry investment, ensuring that the UK remains a competitive environment in which to work is undoubtedly an objective for government. This economic power and its political connections provides a strong negotiating position in relation to government.

In the UK, the pharmaceutical industry is regulated to ensure patient access to safe and effective medication. Kay (2001a, 2001b) argues that the regulatory process has become more formal and rule-based since 1997, and that this has put strain level of trust between industry and government. The regulatory framework covers the drug development process, including clinical trials, the licensing of medicines through the MHRA, the pricing of generic and branded pharmaceuticals, the promotion of medicines, the reporting of adverse events and in recent years regulation has expanded to include decisions on the efficacy of drugs through NICE. In addition to this, within the UK, the ABPI produces a voluntary code of practice dealing with the promotion and marketing of prescription-only medicines. It is administered and enforced through the Prescription Medicines Code of Practice Authority. The Code addresses issues relating to advertising, relationships with professionals, patient groups and the public (ABPI 2006).

Points of Contact Between the DH and Industry

Unsurprisingly governments' interaction with the pharmaceutical industry encompasses more than the DH. For example, the Treasury and the Department of Trade and Industry (DTI) have an interest in securing inward investment, the Home Office deals with issues relating to animal welfare in pharmacological research and the Department of Education and Skills (DfES) works with industry to ensure access to an appropriately skilled workforce. The focus of this chapter is however on interactions and avenues for influence within the DH. The main point of contact is through the department's Industry Branch. Its role is to support the UK pharmaceutical and medical devises industry. In so doing it acts as the industry's principle channel of communication with Government and services regular meetings between industry and Ministers, according to the DH website:

> The overall purpose is to ensure that Government's actions and intentions are understood in the industry and the industry's legitimate concerns are understood and addressed within Government (DH, 2006).

The Pharmaceutical Price Regulation Scheme

As the lead in the negotiations with the pharmaceutical industry on the price the NHS pays for branded-medicines, the Industry Branch manages and administers the Pharmaceutical Price Regulatory Scheme (PPRS). This agreement is negotiated every five years between the pharmaceutical industry represented by the ABPI and the government. The objectives of the PPRS are to:

- secure the provision of safe and effective medicines for the NHS at reasonable prices;
- promote a strong and profitable pharmaceutical industry capable of such sustained research and development expenditure as should lead to the future availability of new and improved medicines;
- encourage the efficient and competitive development and supply of medicines to pharmaceutical markets in this and other countries (DH, 1999).

These objectives point to an inherent dilemma for the DH in negotiations it must decide where the trade-off between value of money and industry support lies. In effect the PPRS is a supply-side intervention to control government expenditure on medicines. Currently around 12 percent of the NHS budget is spent on pharmaceuticals. It sets a cap on the profits that industry can make in selling medicines to the NHS, but leaves industry free to determine what they charge for individual brands. This means they are still able to achieve premium prices for newer medicines but only if they reduce the prices of their other products. Although the ABPI negotiates an overall agreement with the DH, each pharmaceutical company is able to interpret it individually. Kay (2001a) argues that under New Labour PPRS negotiations have become contentious. During the talks over the 1999/2004 scheme, discussions were more fraught because government had indicated its goal of pursuing price cuts and taken steps to put this voluntary scheme onto a statutory footing via the 1999 Health Act. The statutory powers were brought in because there were concerns that a small number of companies had begun testing the agreement by increasing prices. Government has yet to use these powers, the flexibility of the voluntary scheme, against the rigidity of a statutory agreement has encouraged industry to commit to a negotiated settlement. In recent years, the DH has sought to open up the transparency of the PPRS process, for example, prior to the discussions for the 2005/2009 scheme, it initiated a public consultation on the scheme. As it stands the PPRS offers advantages for both government and industry, government is able to set a limit on what it is willing to pay for medicines and meet its goal of supporting industry and industry benefits from a relatively stable trading environment and is able to set prices for new medicines as it sees fit (ABPI, 2005).

From the interviews, it was clear that negotiations can lead to tensions between government and industry 'there are times when it [the relationship] is strained particularly around the time of the PPRS' (PS5). However, respondents from the pharmaceutical industry were generally positive about the PPRS, believing that it worked as a mechanism for regulating prices. One industry representative said 'it's a compromise, where industry is happy and government is happy … the worry is if you get rid of PPRS which has worked… it meets its goal in a fairly opaque way, if you throw that out and start again, what do you start with?' (PI2). Yet there was criticism from those within industry that the PPRS was too focussed on with securing short-term savings rather than promoting long-term investment and encouraging innovation.

The future of the PPRS has now been called into question, in early 2007, an OFT review of whether the current scheme is the most effective mechanism for meeting its aims and objectives recommended that it should be reformed in the 2010 round of negotiations. The OFT argued that for some treatment areas such as high cholesterol and blood pressure, the NHS was paying too much for medicines. It recommended that value for money would be better achieved if prices were set according to the clinical and therapeutic benefit for patients, in addition it argued that this system would encourage industry to invest in areas where there were few or no treatments (OFT, 2007). The Government's response (from both the DH and the DTI) to the review is due in summer 2007. Given the criticism of current practices, it is likely that the government will respond positively to the review and promise some revision of the process, although whether there is the stomach to completely revise the scheme and the protracted negotiations that this would require with industry, remains to be seen.

Ensuring Long-term Investment

Concerns about how government reforms such as creation of NICE and the decision to legislate on price control powers would affect the long-term investment decisions by industry led the Chief Executive Officers of the then three remaining UK companies: AstraZeneca, Glaxo Wellcome and SmithKline Beecham to request a meeting in November 1999 with Prime Minister Tony Blair. Keen to assuage industry fears about the future, in early 2000 the Pharmaceutical Industry Competitiveness Taskforce (PICTF) was established. The terms of reference were to:

> bring together the expertise and experience of the industry leaders in the UK with Government policy makers to identify and report to the Prime Minister on the steps that may need to be taken to retain and strengthen the competitiveness of the UK business environment for the innovative pharmaceutical industry (PICTF, 2001: 5).

The DH and industry took joint-responsibility for the secretariat of PICTF, but its focus was beyond health policy and the NHS, for example, it addressed issues relating to the skills base of the workforce, and pressures in the global economy. The taskforce comprised Ministers from the DH, the DTI, DfES and the Home Office along with representatives from industry and the ABPI. In addition representatives from other government departments attended meetings as and when necessary, along with an observer from the Prime Ministers' Policy Office.

Six working groups were established to look at areas which were identified as impacting on UK competitiveness: Developments in the UK market; Intellectual Property Rights; Regulation of medicines licensing; Science-base and biopharmaceuticals; Clinical research; and the wider economic climate (PICTF, 2001). In relation to the NHS, industry argued that in addition to existing limits on GP prescribing, the creation of NICE was another control on the availability of branded-medicines (see below). There was also a desire that industry should have a role in the development and implementation of National Service Frameworks; that the potential for greater use by industry of NHS information, particularly in tracking the efficacy of medicines should be explored; that there was a need for appropriate information on medicines for patients to ensure concordance; and that research opportunites of pharmacogenetics should not be missed (PICTF, 2001).

The taskforce reported in 2001, identifying a number of recommendations for both government and industry to take forward. The report also set out performance indicators to ensure that the UK remained a long-term investment opportunity. It was clear that the taskforce had improved relationships between industry and government, providing an opportunity for a new partnership in taking forward the agenda of both industry and government, the Chief Executive of Astra Zeneca was quoted as saying:

> PICTF has strengthened industry-Government relationships, significantly increased mutual understanding and delivered some valuable outputs (PICTF, 2001: 2).

The benefits of this dialogue was also noted in the interviews, with respondents arguing the process begun by PICTF had helped forge potentially beneficial relationships and begun to restore trust, a civil servant noted:

> I think we learnt that if we have a constructive and open relationship its better for everyone, they recognise and we recognise that there will be issues that we won't agree on … but if we can fight ourselves to a draw … you can progress (PS5).

The report argued that regular high-level dialogue should continue and to this end, the Ministerial Industry Strategy Group (MISG) was established. Again Ministers from a number of departments and senior industry representatives met regularly to ensure that progress against the recommendations of PICTF is being achieved. However, by late 2004 concerns were being raised that there was a danger that the MISG was becoming little more than a 'talking shop' (PI2) and there was a need to develop a more structured process. As a consequence the 'Long-Term Leadership Strategy' was established, which aimed to:

- secure the provision of safe and effective medicines for patients, and to advance healthcare information;
- strengthen the environment for the pharmaceutical industry in Europe;
- improve the efficiency of medicines regulation in the UK and Europe (DH, 2007).

Its work focused on developing partnership working between NHS and industry to ensure the effective use medicines; support the development of similar European-wide strategies aimed at improving competitiveness and finally an assessment of regulatory processes. The group reported in early 2007 and produced a number of recommendations aimed at ensuring that the UK and Europe remains an attractive to inward investment and a continuing dialogue between industry and government. This process is constantly evolving, in early 2007, an extended terms of reference and membership of the MISG was announced (DH, 2007).

The PICTF/MISG/LTLS process has shown that government is willing to ensure that mechanisms are put into place to support industry, unsurprising since this is part of the DH's brief. The Health Select Committee was critical 'government's excessive focus on ensuring the competitiveness of the industry to the disadvantage of the NHS and patients' (HC, 2005: 15). However, it should also be possible to use this process to push the industry's R&D agenda to deal with particular health concerns, this was noted by one industry respondent who after acknowledging much of the agenda is currently pushed by industry said:

> the DH could be coming to us and saying 'diabetes is a huge problem, if you could develop a diabetes drug that meet these criteria we will give it a premium price, we will fast track it', but they aren't doing that, but it has been identified as a potential area (PI2).

External Pressures

So far the evidence suggests that the DH is sympathetic and supportive to industry and they have a productive relationship. Indeed, the majority of interviewees described the relationship between government and industry as being 'close' and 'constructive'. While some interviewees suggested that this had changed little since New Labour came to power, the majority, argued that after initial distrust, both sectors have worked hard to build a good working relationship. However, external pressures have at times threatened this dialogue, this section explores the impact of three key areas, the creation of NICE, the Health Select Committee review of the influence of industry and the activities of other stakeholders in the health policy arena.

The National Institute for Health and Clinical Excellence

In 1999 the special health authority National Institute for Clinical Excellence (now the National Institute for Health and Clinical Excellence – NICE) was established to provide guidance on the use of new and existing medicines, to develop clinical guidelines and to assist with clinical audit in the NHS. The government claimed NICE would help reduce variations in access to medication and treatments across the country, so-called post-code prescribing. NICE assesses the evidence-base for interventions and judges their potential cost-effectiveness and efficacy. Its recommendations can determine whether or not new treatments will be prescribed on the NHS. It is unsurprising therefore that NICE decisions have strained relationships between industry and government. One of its first rulings, against the provision of the flu drug Relenza, led to threats of disinvestment in the UK (MacDonald, 2000). In addition, 'NICE-blight' – the refusal of Primary Care Trusts to provide new interventions before they have been through the NICE process, and the delay in uptake of interventions once approval has been given, has led to criticism of NICE, not just from within industry, but patients' groups, and professionals (HC, 2002; Baggott, 2004).

In recent months industry has shown an increased willingness to challenge the NICE process through litigation. In November 2006 following the rejection by NICE of three drugs developed for the treatment of Alzhemier's disease, the manufacturers of the drugs announced they would be seeking judicial review of the criteria used to measure cost-effectiveness in decision making (Hawkes, 2007). Pressure from industry and patients groups has also led in one instance, to the negotiation of a risk-sharing deal with industry. NICE's refusal to approve Beta Interferon for Multiple Sclerosis because of insufficient evidence of efficacy led the DH to agree a deal where reimbursement would be provided for those patients where the drug was proved to be clinically effective, but the manufacturer would cover costs where no benefit was proven. Interestingly, the OFT (2007) review suggested that a version of this model could be one part of a new mechanism to replace PPRS.

In interview, representatives from the pharmaceutical industry were critical of NICE, although they were aware that assessment of effectiveness was an inherent feature of modern healthcare systems, one representative said 'we accept that regulatory approval is no longer a gateway to use' (PI2). Of particular concern was the ability of companies to provide the type of evidence required for reviews. One respondent say it is 'impossible for any company to have the body of evidence necessary to demonstrate clinical-effectiveness and cost-effectiveness' (PI3). One solution put forward by industry and others (HC, 2005) is the need for earlier dialogue in the drug development process to discuss the needs of regulators, so that clinical trials could be designed to provide appropriate evidence.

In interview, it was suggested by some industry observers that in recent years NICE has helped moderate the influence of pharmaceutical industry because it must prove the efficacy of new treatments. There is no doubt that industry has directly lobbied government on NICE decisions, however, there are growing concerns that industry is also attempting to influence NICE and government indirectly by surreptitiously supporting lobbying by professionals and patients' groups (Templeton, 2006). For the most part government has backed the independence of NICE rulings – although late last year concerns were raised when Patricia Hewitt seemingly pre-empted a NICE ruling on the breast cancer drug Herceptin. In February 2007, the Health Select Committee announced it was undertaking a second review of NICE, looking in particular at why its decisions were being increasingly challenged, its evaluation and appeals processes (HC, 2007).

Health Select Committee

In June 2004 the Parliamentary Health Committee announced that it planned to investigate the influence of the pharmaceutical industry, its terms of reference were to:

> Undertake an inquiry into the influence of the pharmaceutical industry on health policies, health outcomes and future health priorities and needs. The inquiry will focus, in particular, on the impact of the industry on: drug innovation; the conduct of medical research; the provision of drug information and promotion; professional and patient education; regulatory review of drug safety and efficacy; and product evaluation, including assessments of value for money (HC, 2005: 9)

This was the first inquiry into the pharmaceutical industry since 1914, and collected oral evidence from over 50 experts and over 100 written memoranda (HC, 2005). The committee reported in March 2005, and its recommendations covered issues relating to drug development, medical research, regulation, access to medicines, and relationships with the public, professionals and government. It argued that 'at almost every level of NHS care provision the pharmaceutical industry shapes the agenda and the practice of medicine' (HC, 2005: 44). In particular the report was critical of government's failure to establish appropriate regulatory systems to tackle the short-comings of industry in particular the lack of innovation in drug development, influence over other stakeholders, poor reporting of iatrogenic affects and the increasing medicalisation of society. In addition, the review recommended that the industry sponsorship should be moved to the DTI and that a national policy framework for drug development should be established (HC, 2005).

A number of interviewees commented that the review caused friction at its outset. Following the announcement of the special advisors to the committee, all considered vocal critics of industry practices, the ABPI successfully lobbied government to include an advisor who would be more sympathetic to the industry's agenda. Interviewees from industry were critical of the way the review had been established, arguing that it was inherently biased – one talked of the committee looking for the smoking-gun. Yet the report was more critical of regulatory processes than industry practices, arguing that they should be tightened to control industry influence. One stakeholder said 'the people who came out worse were the MHRA … the pharmaceutical companies came out surprising unscathed' (PS6). Indeed, both industry representatives and stakeholders were generally positive about the outcome of the review. One industry respondent said 'we agreed with three quarters of the recommendations' (PI4).

In interview that both industry representatives and observers recognised that the report had had an impact on industry. In particular on the ABPI Code of Practice which was under review at the time the report was published, was considered to be a stronger document as a consequence. One interviewee said 'it held a mirror up to industry' (PI2) and another said 'it certainly focused the mind [of industry] and ensured that rigorous new code was agreed with an unwritten threat that if the industry didn't get its act together a statutory one would soon follow' (PI3). Interviewees also argued that the review had done little to damage relationships between industry and the DH, since 'both were in the dock' (PI3). Indeed some recommendations had identified areas where government needed to work closer with industry, one interviewee said it had influenced the Long-Term Leadership Strategy because 'a lot of the recommendations are around regulation and that's one of the reason the government was keen to set up the regulatory group' (PI2).

In response to the review (DH, 2005) government signalled that it was prepared to act on a number of recommendations, although number were rejected, including the split of the sponsorship function from the DH, so the tension of balancing interests and making trade-offs remains (cf. Abraham, 2006; Collier, 2006). An industry representative welcomed the decision not to split the function arguing that 'if they had no requirement to think about industry policy and industry you would get an increasingly procurement mind-set' (PI2). Yet other stakeholders were concerned arguing that the interests of industry would always have the upper hand in any negotiations and agreements between DH and industry.

The Broader Health Policy Arena

The activities of other healthcare stakeholders also influence the relationship between government and industry. For example, in recent years new stakeholders, groups representing the interests of health service users, have become increasingly incorporated into the health policy process (Baggott, Allsop and Jones, 2005). Some of these groups may be potential allies in the policy process, with both sectors sharing an interest in ensuring patients have access to medicines, others particularly those set up as a consequence of adverse events are increasingly challenging industry practices (Allsop, Jones and Baggott, 2005). For those groups who choose to work with industry, in particular those willing to accept funding there have been growing disquiet among policy makers that these links are opaque. In particular, the concern that groups may be used to push the industry's agenda and damage their own reputation and ability to claim independence (Which, 2003; Templeton, 2006). Industry's revised code of practice now says that industry must published details of the financial support they give to groups (ABPI, 2006).

Opinion formers such as the media can also be influential, Kay (2001a) shows how press reports added to the tension in the debates around the 1999 PPRS. One industry representative suggested that criticisms from the media have prompted industry to be more transparent. Media coverage is also used as a tactic by other groups in the policy process, particularly around issues on access to medicines and NICE rulings.

Finally, interviewees also talked about how events at international level, particularly the European Union (EU), were also having an impact at national level. Regulatory convergence particularly over the licensing of medicines, the EU High-Level Pharmaceutical Forum which aims to encourage investment in the Europe and EU discussions on direct to consumer information were identified as issues that were now or could in the future have an impact on pharmaceutical policy in the UK.

Conclusions

Relationships between government and industry have clearly improved since the impasse in the late-1990s when government plans for NICE and the PPRS had caused friction. Since then government has increasingly responded to industry's agenda, working with it to secure long-term investment. However, this may be less to do with the power of industry than with government's desire to ensure that the UK retains one of its gold-standard industries, as a civil servant said 'we all know we could get lower prices, but there is an industrial policy [to be considered] here' (PS4).

Given the apparent willingness of government to support industry interests, few interviewees actually regarded the pharmaceutical sector as the most powerful influence on health policy. Those that did argued that the financial power of industry meant that it was able to call the shots. However, other interviewees argued that professional interests, in particular doctors, still carried more weight in the policy process and highlighted the role of the Treasury in setting the policy agenda. Industry respondents argued that while government was willing to listen to their concerns, it was prepared to take on industry, citing price cuts imposed by the PPRS and NICE rulings as areas where industry had been unable to get its own way.

References

ABPI (Association of the British Pharmaceutical Industry) (2005), 'Understanding the 2005 PPRS Industry Briefing', London, ABPI.

ABPI (Association of the British Pharmaceutical Industry) (2006), Code of Practice.

Abraham, J. (2005), 'Regulating the drugs industry transparently', *British Medical Journal*, **331**, 528–29.

Allsop, J., Jones, K. and Baggott, R.(2004), 'Health consumer groups: A new social movement?' *Sociology of Health and Illness*, **26**(6) 737–56.

Baggott, R. (2004), Health and Health Care in Britain (3rd edn), Palgrave Macmillan, Basingstoke.

Baggott, R., Allsop, J. and Jones, K. (2005), *Speaking for Patients and Carers: Health Consumer Groups and the Policy Process*, Palgrave Macmillan, Basingstoke.

Busfield, J. (2003), 'Globalisation and the pharmaceutical industry revisited', *International Journal of Health Services*, **33**(3) 681–605.

Collier, J. (2006), 'Big Pharma and Government', *The Lancet*, **365**(9505) 97–98.

DH (Department of Health) (1999), The Pharmaceutical Price Regulation Scheme, TSO, London.

DH (Department of Health) (2005), Government response to the Health Committee's report on the influence of the pharmaceutical industry, (Cm 6655), DoH, London.

DH (Department of Health) (2006), Ministry Industry Strategy Group, www.dh.gov.uk, (consulted Oct. 2006).

DH (Department of Health) (2007), Ministerial Industry Strategy Group, DoH, London.

Grant, W. (1989), Pressure Groups Politics and Democracy in Britain, Phillip Allan, London.

Hawkes, N. (17 November 2007), 'Secrecy over NHS drug rationing faces court challenge', *The Times*, 10.

HC (Health Committee) (2002), National Institute for Clinical Excellence, Second Report Session 2001/02, HC 515–I, TSO, London.

HC (Health Committee) (2005), The Influence of the Pharmaceutical Industry, Fourth Report Session 2004/2005 HC 42-I, TSO, London.

HC (Health Committee) (2007), The National Institute for Health and Clinical Excellence, www.parliament.uk, (consulted Feb. 2007).

HM Treasury (2004), Advancing long-term prosperity: Economic reform in an enlarged Europe, www.hm-treasury.gov.uk, (consulted Jan. 2007).

Herxheimer, A. (2003), 'Relationships Between the Pharmaceutical Industry and Patients Organisations', *British Medical Journal*, **326**, 1208–1210.

Kay, A. (2001a), 'New Labour on drugs: The changing relationship between government and the pharmaceutical industry', *Political Quarterly*, 322–328.

Kay, A. (2001b), 'Pharmaceutical policy in the UK', *Public Money & Management*, Oct–Dec, 51–54.

McDonald, R. (2000), 'Just say no? Drugs, politics and the UK National Health Service', *Policy & Politics*, **28**(4) 563–76.

Moran, M. (1999), Governing the healthcare state: A comparative study of the United Kingdom, United State and Germany, Manchester University Press, Manchester.

Moynihan, R., Heath, I. and Henry, D. (2002), 'Selling sickness, the pharmaceutical industry and disease mongering', *British Medical Journal*, **324**, 886–891.

O'Donovan, O. and Glavanis-Grantham, K. (2005), Patients' Organisations in Ireland, Challenging Capitalist Biomedicine? Final Report to the Royal Irish Academy Third Sector Research Programme, University of Cork, Cork.

OFT (2007), OFT report recommends reform to UK drug pricing scheme, OFT Press Release 29/07, OFT, London.

PICTF (2001), Pharmaceutical Industry Competitiveness Task Force: Final Report, DoH, London.

Pollock, A. (2004), NHS Plc., Verso, London.

Templeton, S. (3 December 2006), 'Health charities get 'covert' aid from drug firms', *Sunday Times*, 6.

Toynbee, P. (24 October 2006), 'Comment and Debate', *The Guardian*, 33.

Which? (April 2003), 'Who's injecting the cash?', *Which*, 24–25.

Chapter 14

The New General Practice Contract and Reform of Primary Care in the UK

Alison Hann

Recent political and organisational changes in the UK NHS have created shifting contexts for the delivery of primary health care. In England, most interest has been paid to the developing market reforms incorporating patient choice, Choose and Book, payment by results, Foundation Trust status, developing a provider market and practice based purchasing (PbC) – although the supply side reforms in Northern Ireland, Scotland and Wales provide useful comparative context within the UK. However, it is the introduction of the new GMS contract that has had the greatest impact on general practice and continues to have the greatest potential for change – especially when combined with other changes in the English NHS such as the IM&T strategy. The new contract offers a unique experiment in the use of incentives to reward quality through the *Quality and Outcomes Framework* that provides financial rewards to general practices based on a points system of over 150 quality indicators covering clinical, organisational and patient focused aspects of practice (Smith and York, 2004).

This chapter examines the impact of the new GMS (nGMS) contract within the changing organisational and policy context of the English NHS. We begin by outlining the current policy context for the English NHS before moving on to examine the current contractual arrangements for general practice. The next section then discusses the potential impacts on general practice in the UK. The chapter ends by discussing what some of the wider implications of the new contract might be in the UK more generally – particularly within the context of the development of differing health systems in Northern Ireland, Scotland and Wales.

The Policy Context

The aims of the current range of NHS reforms in England are threefold. The first is to incentivise organisational reform through practice based commissioning, patient choice and payment by results. The second aim is to allow greater autonomy at a local level but on a selective basis with decentralisation only afforded to those organisations whose performance (as measured by government measures) is rated highly (such as granting Foundation Trust status to NHS hospitals which are rated as performing well). The third aim is to create a pluralist model of local provision within the public, private and not-for-profit sectors. The purchaser-provider distinction (first created in the 1990s quasi-market) is being extended to allow new market entrants and patient choice policy *requires* patients to be given a choice of 4–5 providers at the point of referral by the GP, one of whom has to be a private/independent organisation – a process built into the new Choose and Book software used to arrange referrals (DoH, 2004, 2005a, 2006). These organisational developments in commissioning and service use provide a rapidly evolving context for general practice within which changes to the GP contract need to be analysed especially as the contract is UK wide while there are different policy and organisational contexts in England, Northern Ireland, Scotland and Wales (Exworthy, 1998; Greer, 2004, 2005).

Changes in primary care also need to be set within the wider health and social care context in the UK. There is an increasing recognition of the need to support self care and informal care (DoH, 2006; Kerr, 2005) with a growing recognition that long term and chronic health problems are not satisfactorily addressed within the UK NHS (Coulter, 2006). In England the recent White Papers have stressed the importance of self care and the role of the NHS in supporting it, the need to build peoples skills for preventing ill health and highlighted the need to support people with long-term conditions to manage independently (DoH, 2004, 2005b, 2006). People with chronic disease are more likely to be users of the health system, accounting for some 80 per cent of all GP consultations while as much as 40 per cent of general practice consultations are for minor ailments that could be taken care of by people themselves (DoH, 2005c; Wilson et al., 2005). While there is widespread public support for self care recent surveys suggest that despite a well established structure for managing individual care through general practice, the primary health care team and PCT co-ordination, the NHS is poor at providing support for self care (Coulter, 2006; DoH, 2004, 2005d; Ellins and Coulter, 2005; Wilson et al., 2005).

Public health activities have also been prioritised through a system of changes to the GMS contract and introduction of financial incentives. The need to develop a stronger public health approach in primary care has long been recognised but despite changes to GP contracts in 1990 and making public health a key objective of primary care organisations from the mid 1990s developments have been limited and the most recent Healthcare Commission annual report highlights the lack of investment in, and low priority given to public health (Healthcare Commission 2006, Peckham and Exworthy 2003, Peckham 2003).

General practice in the UK also faces a number of other challenges resulting from changes in the workforce, greater pressure to apply evidence based medicine and treatment protocols and meet centrally set targets. It is into this complex context that the new contract has been introduced. In addition access to primary care in the UK has fundamentally changed in recent years with the introduction of NHS Direct (24 hour telephone/internet advice service), walk-in centres and a growing private provision of general practice, CAM and physiotherapy and counselling services (Peckham, 2004, 2006). These challenges are not unrecognised by the profession and the need for general practice to respond to social change was the topic of a Royal College of General Practitioners working group on the future of general practice (Wilson et al., 2006).

The New GMS Contract

In 2004 the new general medical services contract was introduced in the UK. The contract marked a major change in the way GPs are contracted with the NHS. Under the old contract GP principals held an individual contract that, despite changes in substance remained based on the original contract established in 1948. GP incomes were made up from a mixture of funding for registered patients, undertaking specific activities and support for practice development such as nursing and administration staff (Moon and North, 2000). The new GMS contract was developed from pilots of new contractual forms introduced in the late 1990s under Primary Medical Services (PMS) designed to stimulate innovation in practice (Riley et al., 2003, Meads et al., 2003).

The main principles of the new contract are:

- A shift from individual GP to practice based contracts,
- Contracts based around workload management with core and enhanced service levels,
- A reward structure based on a new quality and outcomes framework an annual assessments,
- An expansion of primary care services,
- Modernisation of practice infrastructure (especially IT systems).

Aspects of the new contractual arrangements for general practice that are less discussed includes Personal Medical Services (PMS), Alternative Provider Medical Services (APMS) and Specialist Provider Medical Services (SPMS) contracts. PMS originated in 1996 to encourage innovation in structure and services in general practice and about one third of practices held a PMS contract in 2005. While there has been some innovation with a greater emphasis placed on multi-professional models with less GP involvement they have not, as yet significantly challenged the dominant general practice model of a small team of GPs supported by other staff. The introduction of salaried GPs and nurse practitioners were identified as key new approaches there has been little encroachment on the organisation of practices and nurse led practices or nurse practitioners remain scarce – only nine nurse led practices have been developed and growth in the numbers of salaried GPs in non PMS and PMS practices is similar (Sibbald et al., 2000). Structural barriers to non GP provided practice remain engrained in professional guidelines and statutory responsibilities for prescribing and patient care (Houghton, 2002). Importantly, the experience of PMS paved the way for the introduction of the new GMS contract (Smith et al., 2005).

Contracts under APMS and SPMS are much rarer and while the opportunity to develop new forms of primary care practice exists, few contracts have been let. These variations on the GMS contract were introduced by the government to encourage NHS commissioners to explore alternative organisational models of primary care, particularly from the independent and private sectors but local hostility has limited success. In Derbyshire an APMS was let to United Healthcare but local residents have forced a judicial review of the PCTs decision and the process has now been started again but with three local residents sitting patient/public representatives on the commissioning panels. Medical professional groups also remain generally hostile to the encroachment of large private companies in general practice. SPMS contracts have also been used to develop local primary care services but again their use has been limited. To date the use of such contracts has been to develop specialist private services (nurses and therapists working in the community in Surrey are proposing to use SPMS to establish a limited company) or to establish new formal relationships in virtual organisations to deliver care in well defined circumstances (e.g. integrated care services in Epsom and in North Bradford and drug abuse and long term care services) (CSIP 2006).

Quality and Outcomes Framework

While there are a number of controversial aspects to the new contract, the Quality Outcomes Framework (QOF) has generated most debate and discussion. QOF provides financial incentives for general practices to meet a range of clinical, organisational and patient experience criteria. It is a voluntary system that practices opt into and is worth approximately £125,000 per annum for a practice if maximum points are achieved. Practices accumulate points for reaching set targets and then receive income for each point achieved (Smith and York, 2004). In 2004/2005, the first year of operation, 222 practices (2.6 per cent) achieved the maximum number of points (1050) with the average score being 958.7 points although nearly half of all practices in England (4243) achieved a score between 1000 and 1050. The QOF framework underwent changes into the second year to expand the range of clinical areas and place more emphasis on health promotion activities. The outcome for 2005/2006 showed that practices had improved their performance across the areas identified in QOF (see QOF website at: http://www.ic.nhs.uk/services/qof) but little research has examined the impact of the use of such incentives on the overall process of patient care in general practice – particularly the extent to which the use of financial targets alter local practice. Similar improvements in achieving standards occurred in Wales and Scotland suggesting that despite differing institutional frameworks and policy environments general practice has responded to QOF incentives in a similar way across the UK. Discussion are currently underway between the British Medical Association (negotiating on behalf of GPs) and the Department of Health on focusing QOF more on self care support and interventions to reduce demand in primary care.

Two aspects of QOF are of interest. The first is the use of financial targets to change behaviour and second the impact of target systems on practice. While the QOF framework is still fairly new there is some indication that both these factors are likely to be of increasing importance in the development of primary care services. Marshall and Harrison (2005) have suggested that use of targets and financial incentives may have unintended consequences on practitioner behaviour such as goal displacement and rule following leading to the 'crowding out' of and reduction in focus on non-incentivised tasks. Thus areas of clinical activity not included within QOF may become seen to be less important. Studies have also found that financial reward is not necessarily the main incentive for practitioners to engage in quality improvement (Spooner et al., 2001) and while targets clearly deliver changes in behaviour may lead to goal misplacement in which rule following becomes the means to the end (Harrison and Smith, 2004). In terms of impact on the practice, the fact that practices have universally opted in to the QOF process demonstrates that financial payments are a key incentive to adopt new processes. However, embedding QOF in practices has implications for both organisational and clinical processes which are discussed later in this paper. One immediate requirement to opt in to QOF is, however, the need for IT systems and the ability of practices to run the relevant software to collect data.

The development and introduction of IT systems to 'manage' QOF has been central to new approaches to patient management in general practice. There is a need to collect data to record activity against the QOF criteria and practitioner prompt/reminder programmes are also widely used. This is where GPs are prompted to ensure that patients have had a variety of tests and screening at each visit and practitioners have to ensure they record data on visits so that this can be used to demonstrate that QOF targets and being achieved and that data can be collected to produce QOF returns at the end of the year. This central role of IM&T systems has, however, had other effects on clinical management processes in general practice as systems are developed to respond to the changes in QOF itself.

Implications For Practice

What impact will these changes in the GMS contract, and introduction of PbC have when combined with the wider reforms within the English NHS? Wilson et al (2006) have suggested that there are four broad areas upon which the performance of primary care, and general practice specifically, should be measured. These are equity, quality of clinical care, responsiveness to patients and efficiency. UK general practice scores highly on these criteria but concerns about lack of support for self care (DoH, 2005c, 2005d), poor support for people with long-term conditions (Coulter, 2006) and the fact that inequalities in health at a primary care level persist (Wilson et al., 2006) raise questions about whether general practice will retain this strong position.

To date general practice in the UK has scored very highly in comparisons of equity of access (Blendon et al., 2002) although the inequity in the distribution of GPs continues to worsen with fewer GPs per registered population in more deprived areas (Hann and Gravelle, 2004). Research on financial incentives for public health found that financial reward for practices bore no relation to local need and recent research in Scotland found that there are small inequalities between practices in service provision for simple monitoring interventions, but larger inequalities for diagnostic, outcome and treatment measures (Langham et al., 1995, McClean et al., 2006). In addition, QOF may skew practices to completing labour intensive interventions (such as the screening and treatment for hypertension) rather than interventions with greater potential for health gain (such as ACE in heart failure) they receive higher financial reward (Fleetcroft and Cookson 2006). Early analysis of QOF also suggests there is a correlation between exception reporting (the exclusion of patients from reported figures for reasons such as patients consistently refusing to attend interviews, patients too frail, lack of service) and social deprivation indices (Sigfrid et al., 2006; Galvin, 2006).

While progress on improving clinical care in general practice has been substantial there are still gaps with a wide variation in the quality of care for different patients (Seddon et al., 2001). Major successes have been in areas where targets have been set or additional resources have been provided (Campbell et al., 2003, 2005). Given this the QOF process should lead to improvements in clinical care as it provides targets associated with additional funding. There is emerging evidence, though, that the use of the QOF framework is changing relationships in practices with responses to changes in QOF becoming primarily a technical problem requiring attention to design of information systems to rationalise practice and collect the relevant data rather than being addressed as a clinical issue for guiding practitioner practice (Checkland, 2006). What impact this will have on the quality of care is not clear at the present time but challenges the concept of individualised care. In addition, the numbers of practitioners dealing with the care of individual patients due to meeting 24/48 hour targets and increasing range of people involved raises questions about continuity of care and clinical quality.

The third area of performance is responsiveness to patients. UK general practice enjoys a high level of patient satisfaction although patients express dissatisfaction about their levels of involvement in decisions about their care (Health Care Commission, 2005; Wilson et al., 2006). High satisfaction may be influenced by more general factors such as location, relatively easy access, longer consultation times and improved use of the wider primary health care team (Wilson et al., 2006). Responsiveness also includes the appropriate application of resources in accordance with need. International comparison demonstrates that the UK NHS system has reduced health costs and that the wide access to general practice services reduces demand for specialist, hospital care (Starfield, 1998; Roberts and May, 1998). Data from QOF has identified that practices are undertaking more activity – whether this is actual or better measured is perhaps open to debate and there are concerns about the impact of QOF on equity. The introduction of PBC may help to drive further cost efficiencies in patient care although the evidence to support significant cost savings in previous primary care led purchasing has been equivocal (Smith et al., 2005). How far PCTs can maintain a co-ordinated approach across practices to reduce inequities and allocative inefficiencies remains to be seen – particularly as patient choice will increase uncertainty in local health care systems.

The increasing emphasis on self care and public health should mean that that general practice, as the most local and universally accessed part of the NHS, plays a key role in these areas. The development of QOF criteria focusing on public health measures and clinical care for people with CHD, diabetes etc represents a shift towards trying to incentivise practices to specific activities. However, the steep increase in GP earnings and questions about actual increases in activity have been highlighted in the media and there has also been criticism from within the nursing profession that while pay rises were meant to reward additional work in the practice the main group of staff undertaking these wider health promotion and patient support roles are in fact nurses, not GPs (Amicus/CPHVA 2006). The contract raises important questions about the internal relationships within practices about the appropriate staff mix to provide the types of services practices are being encouraged to develop and also whether processes (for meeting QOF targets for example) have become more important drivers in general practice than clinical expertise. Early evidence suggests that while there is potential in these contract mechanisms to change practice behaviour and work process the current direction would seem to be one that is creating more techno-bureaucratic approaches to patient care. PCTs and other health care purchasers have not yet sufficiently used the flexibilities that the contract provides to explore new models of primary care and the focus on private provision may be unhelpful as it has led to conflict. In fact, most private primary care provision has been developed by GPs and models of care are dominated by traditional models of general practice which on the face of emerging evidence have not been particularly successful at addressing long term care needs of patients or addressing key public health problems in local communities (Coulter, 2006; Kai and Drinkwater, 2003).

Finally there are tensions evolving in the system between competing demands and targets. Patient choice and the Choose and Book system focus attention on responsiveness to choices about location of secondary care. However, recent concerns about funding and the need for PCTs as strategic purchasers to manage demand has seen an increase in the use of central referral centres sitting between the GP and the provider. In addition there have been concerns about the NHS IM&T systems and take up of Choose and Book has been slow with many GPs still not using the system (Pothier, 2006).

Conclusion

The use of the financial incentives in QOF to change practice has been shown to work and it is leading to improvements in clinical care across the UK – generating considerable international interest. The more difficult assessment is whether this produces the right improvements or in fact the best value improvements. QOF may actually discriminate against practices in deprived areas reducing their ability to develop the kinds of organisational systems necessary to tackle problems associated with deprived populations as smaller practices in deprived areas do less well than larger practices in affluent areas and that it is the financial reward for better organisational systems that brings increased payments (Wang et al., 2006). Two points that are highly relevant are the need for good organisational structures and processes in family practice for a QOF system to operate (and for practices to gain most) and concerns about the distortion of payments to more affluent areas away from more deprived areas creating further disincentives for practitioners to provide services in less affluent places. The emerging differences between the English, Northern Ireland, Scottish and Welsh NHS systems provides a unique observatory for examining how wider health system context affects the same general practice incentive scheme.

The nGMS and QOF will continue to develop within a changing landscape. In England the development of PbC, pluralist provision, expansion of self care and extension of private providers provides an ever more complex health system. As yet we have not seen a substantial expansion of private provision in the primary care arena and the dominant private model remains the traditional GP model – building on the position of GP as an independent practitioner. Recent announcements to use the APMS and SPMS to extend private provider approaches may change this but challenging dominant models of general practice, that also enjoy high levels of public support, will be difficult. In Wales and Scotland the focus is less on the role of general practice with more central direction and a concern about performance (especially in Wales). In Scotland planned re-organisation of services is largely at a hospital level although the development of local community health and social care partnerships provides a new focus on primary care.

Ultimately though changes in the UK system do not undermine, and in many ways continue to underpin the inter-disciplinary team approach of primary medical. The new contract structures and emphasis on self care, public health etc are key elements of policy but the GP model remains central in these developments and while local funders (such as PCTs) have the potential to develop new innovative models of care using new contractual structures, to date little has been done to do this. How far private and not-for-profit providers are willing to enter such a market remains to be seen – even with government encouragement. To date it is mainly companies run by GPs offering services similar to traditional general practice and perhaps for these reasons they have not been challenged by local professional committees. However, with governments in NI, Scotland and Wales focusing their attention on wider systems issues the impact of the new GMS contract and QOF may go overlooked and there will be a continuing tension between attempts to address systems for self care and supporting people with long term conditions and the incentives of QOF. Whether such tensions can be ironed out through changes in the QOF system itself so that rewards mirror more accurately areas of activity that need to be developed remains to be seen. There are also questions to be explored about how QOF may change the relationship between general practice and the patient. Consultations may become more driven by the demands of QOF or GMS contract targets and the routinisation of specific actions driven by incentive systems rather than the expressed (and sometimes more obscure) needs of the patient. There is little research in this area at the present time but one is for sure – for policy analysts and health researchers the devolved UK NHS provides a unique policy learning laboratory with four system models emerging but with the common feature of the GMS contract and QOF.

References

Amicus/CPHVA (2006), 'Practice nurses get '10 per cent of top GPs pay' but do 50 per cent of the work', (Press release), Amicus/CPHVA, London.

Care Services Improvement Partnership (CSIP) (2006), *Developing Community Hospitals: Models of Ownership*, Department of Health, London.

Checkland, K. (September 2006), 'Collecting data or shaping practice? Evidence from case studies in general practice about the impact of technology associated with the new GMS contract', PSA Annual Health Group Conference, Oxford.

Coulter, A. (2006), *Engaging Patients in Their Healthcare*, Picker Institute Europe, Oxford.

Davies, M. and Elwyn, G. (2006), Referral management centres: Promising innovations or Trojan horses? *British Medical Journal*, **332**, 844–46.

Department of Health (2004), *Choosing Health*, TSO, London.

Department of Health (2005a), Creating a Patient-led NHS: Delivering the NHS Improvement Plan DoH, London.

Department of Health (2005b), *Independence Well-being and Choice*, TSO, London.

Department of Health (2005c), *Self Care – A Real Choice, Self Care Support – A Real Option*, DoH, London.

Department of Health (2005d), *Public Attitudes to Self Care: Baseline Survey*, DoH, London.

Department of Health (2006), *Our Health, Our Care, Our Say*, Cm.,TSO, London.

Ellins, J. and Coulter, A. (2005), *How engaged are people in their health care? Findings of a national telephone survey*, The Health Foundation, London.

Exworthy, M. (1998), 'Primary care in the UK: Understanding the dynamics of devolution', Health and Social Care in the Community, **9**(5) 266–278.

Fleetcroft, R. and Cookson, R. (2006), 'Do incentive payments in the new NHS contract for primary care reflect likely population health gains?' *Journal of Health Services Research and Policy*, **11**(1) 27–31.

Galvin, R. (2006), 'Pay-For-Performance: Too Much Of A Good Thing? A Conversation With Martin Roland', *Health Affairs*, **25**, 412–419.

Greer, S. (2004), *Four Way Bet: How devolution has led to Four Different Models for the NHS*, The Constitution Unit, UCL, London.

Greer, S. (2005), 'Territorial politics and health policy: UK health policy in comparative perspective', Manchester University Press, Manchester.

Guthrie, B., McLean, G., and Sutton, M. (2006), Workload and reward in the Quality and Outcomes Framework of the 2004 general practice contract, *British Journal of General Practice*, **Nov**, 836–841.

Healthcare Commission (2006), *State of Healthcare 2006*, Healthcare Commission. London.

House of Commons (2006), *Public Expenditure on Health and Personal Social Services 2006*, House of Commons, London.

Kai, J. and Drinkwater, C. (eds) (2003), *Primary Care in Urban Disadvantaged Communities*, Radcliffe Medical Press, Oxford.

Kerr D. (2005), Building a Health Service Fit For The Future, Edinburgh, Scottish Executive.

Langham, S., Gillam, S. and Thorogood, M. (1995), 'The carrot, the stick and the general practitioner: how have changes in financial incentives affected health promotion activity in general practice?', *British Journal of General Practice*, **45**, 665–668.

Lipman, T. (2006), 'Singing from the same QOF hymn sheet: stairway to heaven or mephisto waltz?' *British Journal of General Practice*, **Nov**, 819–820.

McClean, G., Sutton, M. and Guthrie, B. (2006), 'Deprivation and quality of primary care services: evidence for persistence of the inverse care law from the UK Quality and Outcomes Framework', *Journal of Epidemiology and Community Health* **60**(11) 917–922.

Marshall, M., and Smith, P. (2003), Rewarding results: using financial incentives to improve quality, *Quality and Safety in Health Care*, **12**, 397–398.

Meads, G., Riley, A.J., Harding, G., and Carter, Y.H. (2004), 'Personal medical services: Local organisational developments', *Primary Health Care Research Development*, **5**(3) 193–201.

Peckham, S (1997) UK general practice fundholding: could it work in Canada? *Canadian Family Physician* **43**, 1–7.

Peckham S. (2003), 'Improving local health', in Dowling, B. and Glendinning, C., *The New Primary Care: Modern, Dependable, Successful?* Open University Press, Buckingham.

Peckham, S. (2004), What choice implies for primary care, *British Journal of Health Care Management*, **10**(7) 210–213.

Peckham, S. (2006), 'The changing context of primary care', *Public Finance and Management*, **6**(4).

Peckham, S., and Exworthy, M. (2003), *Primary Care in the UK: Policy, Organisation and Management*, Basingstoke: Palgrave/MacMillan.

Peckham, S., Exworthy, M., Powell, M. and Greener, I. (2005), *Decentralisation as an Organisational Model for Health Care in England*, Report to NCCSDO.

Pothier, D.D., Awad, Z., and Tierney, P. (2006), 'Choose and Book', in 'ENT, The GP perspective', *Journal of Laryngology and Otology.*

RCGP (2006), *Profile of General Practitioners*, Information Sheet, RCGP, London.

Riley, A.J., Harding, G., Meads, G., Underwood, A.R., and Carter, Y.H. (2003), 'An evaluation of personal medical services pilots: The times they are a changin', *Journal of Interprofessional Care*, **17**(2) 127–139.

Roberts, E., and May, N. (1998), Can primary care and community based models of emergency care substitute for the hospital accident and emergency department? *Health Policy*, **44**, 191–214.

Sibbald, B., Petchey, R., Gosden, T., Leese, B., and Williams, J. (2000), Salaried GPs in PMS pilots: Impact on recruitment, retention, workload, quality of care and cost, in *National Evaluation of First Wave NHS Personal Medical Services Pilots: Integrated Interim Report from Four Research Projects*, Manchester, NPCRDC.

Sigfrid, L.A., Turner, C., Crook, D., and Ray, S. (2006), 'Using the UK primary care Quality and Outcomes Framework to audit health care equity: Preliminary data on diabetes management', *Journal of Public Health*, **28**(3) 221–225.

Smith, J., Ham, C., and Parker, H. (2005), *To market, to market: what future for primary care?* University of Birmingham, Health Services Management Centre, Birmingham.

Smith, P., and York, N. (2004), 'Quality incentives: The case of UK general practitioners', *Health Affairs*, **23**(3) 112–118.

Spurgeon, P., Hicks, C., Field, S., and Barwell, F. (2005), 'The new GMS contract: Impact and implications for managing the changes', *Health Services Management Research*, **18**, 75–85.

Starfield, B. (1998), *Primary Care: Balancing Health Needs, Services and Technology*, Oxford University Press, New York.

Wang, Y., O'Donnell, C.A., Mackay, D.F., and Watt, G.C.M. (2006), 'Practice size and quality attainment under the new GMS contract', *British Journal of General Practice*, **Nov**, 830–835.

Wilson, T., Buck, D., and Ham, C. (2005), 'Rising to the challenge: Will the NHS support people with long term conditions?', *British Medical Journal*, **330**, 657–661.

Index